JN277636

実践・看護の英会話

Everyday English for International Nurses

Joy Parkinson
Chris Brooker

西村月満／平井清子／和治元義博 訳

英和対訳

南雲堂

CHURCHILL LIVINGSTONE
An imprint of Elsevier Limited

Everyday English for International Nurses
A guide to working in the UK

ISBN 0 443 07399 6

©2004, Elsevier Limited. All rights reserved.

First published 2004

The right of Joy Parkinson and Chris Brooker to be identified as authors of this work has been asserted by them in accordance with the Copyright, Designs and Patents Act 1988.

No Part of this publication may be reproduced, stored in a retrieval system, or transmitted in any form or by any means, electronic, mechanical, photocopying, recording or otherwise, without either the prior permission of the publishers or a licence permitting restricted copying in the United Kingdom issued by the Copyright Licensing Agency Ltd, 90 Tottenham Court Road, London W1T 4LP, UK.
Permissions may be sought directly from Elsevier's Health Sciences Right Department in Philadelphia, USA: (+1) 215 238 7869, fax:(+1) 215 238 2239, e-mail: healthpermissions@elsevier.com. You may also complete your request on-line via the Elsevier Science homepage (http://www.elsevier.com), by selecting 'Customer Support' and them 'Obtaining Permissions'.

Japanese edition is published by Nan'un-do Co., Ltd.
This edition of portions of **Everyday English for International Nurses 9780443073991** by **Joy Parkinson, BA and Chris Brooker, BSc, MSc, RGN, SCM, RNT** is published by arrangement with Elsevier Limited through Elsevier Japan KK.

Note
Medical knowledge is constantly changing. As new information becomes available, changes in treatment, procedures, equipment and the use of drugs become necessary. The authors/contributors and the publishers have taken care to ensure that the information given in this text is accurate and up to date. However, readers are strongly advised to confirm that the information, especially with regard to drug usage, complies with current legislation and standards of practice.

はじめに

　あらゆる分野においてグローバル化が進む現在、医療の世界においても、実質的世界共通語となっている英語でコミュニケーションを行う能力の必要性が高まってきています。例えば、日本在住の外国人の方々に医療を提供する場合、あるいは日本人が外国で医療を受ける場合、また最近は日本の高度な医療を受けるために外国人が来日する医療ツアーも行われ、いずれの場合も医療者と患者のコミュニケーションは英語で行われることが多くなっています。

　本書は、このような社会状況を背景として、さまざまな医療の場における看護師と患者の会話を英和対訳で紹介し、加えて医療用語の同義表現や略語も多数紹介することにより、看護学生や看護師だけでなく、広く医療従事者、医療通訳者、医療翻訳者、医療英語教育者の方々の参考とすることを目的に出版されました。

　原著 *Everyday English for International Nurses*（2004）は全11章からなり、イギリスで看護師として仕事をする外国人に向けた著作となっていますが、本書はその中から、日本での出版に最も有用と考えられる第5章「看護におけるコミュニケーション」、第6章中の「病気の医学名と口語名の用語集」、第9章「看護で使用される略語」、第11章「計量単位」、の4章を選び英和対訳といたしました。中心となる「看護におけるコミュニケーション」では、一つ一つの症例における会話から、著者 Parkinson と Brooker が力説する医療におけるコミュニケーション能力の重要性という意味がよく分かります。患者とのたいへん詳しい内容の対話を通じて、その患者のかかえる問題の原因、治療法、解決策などを明らかにしていきます。本書の会話を読むと、是非このような人間的温かみのある看護師のケアを受けたいと感じられることでしょう。本書の会話から、看護における全人的ケアのあり方を知ることができます。本書に紹介されている看護師は、患者を病人というだけでなく、社会生活、家庭生活を営む個人として配慮し、助言を与え、そして患者の尊厳を重んじながらケアを進めています。

　英語面では、第Ⅰ章「看護におけるコミュニケーション」の各ユニットの冒頭にある「Box」という部分によって、読者はそのユニットに関連する医療用語の口語的あるいは俗語的な英語表現が学べるようになっています。また、それに続

く会話において原著者は、しばしば [ ] 内に言い換えを示し、ある一つのことを表現するに際し、日常的表現とやや専門的表現の両方を読者が知ることができるように工夫しています。

　付属のCDには第Ⅰ章の会話部分がイギリス人によって録音されています。イギリス英語に触れながら、発音の確認やリスニング・スキルの向上にぜひ役立てて下さい。

　本書が看護師と患者の間に行なわれる実践的な英会話の例としても、また、イギリスにおける医療のあり方の理解としても、日本の多くの医療関係者の方々の参考となりますよう願っております。

　尚、本書の作成に際し、多大のご助力を賜りました南雲堂営業部岡崎まち子氏、並びに同社編集部加藤敦氏に、心より感謝申し上げます。

　最後に、翻訳には細心の注意をもって取り組みましたが、思いがけない考え違いもあろうかと存じます。皆さまの忌憚ないご指摘を賜ることができましたら幸いです。

訳者一同

　凡例

　（　）＝ 原文にある（　）をそのまま訳したもの
　〔　〕＝ 訳者による補足
　[　]　＝ 主に会話例文中において原著者が口語的表現を説明したもの

Contents

I Communication in nursing
看護におけるコミュニケーション

Unit 1	Introduction はじめに		8
Unit 2	Getting started 会話の開始		10
Unit 3	Breathing 呼吸		28
	Case history 1	Dyspnoea: Mr and Mrs Ryan 呼吸困難：ライアン氏とライアン夫人	
Unit 4	Communicating 意思の疎通		38
	Case history 2	Speech problems due to a stroke: Mrs Egbewole 脳卒中による言語障害：エグベウォゥル夫人	
	Case history 3	Poor hearing and tinnitus: Mr Sandford 聴力障害と耳鳴り：サンドフォード氏	
Unit 5	Safety and preventing accidents 安全と事故防止		50
	Case history 4	A scald: Mrs Kaur （熱湯による）やけど：カウア夫人	
	Case history 5	Instructions on the use of drugs: Mr Anderson 服薬指導：アンダーソン氏	
Unit 6	Mobility 運動能力		60
	Case history 6	Rheumatoid arthritis: Ms Wayne 関節リウマチ：ウェインさん	
	Case history 7	Parkinson's disease: Mr Lajowski パーキンソン病：ラジャウスキ氏	
Unit 7	Eating and drinking 飲食		74
	Case history 8	Loss of appetite and weight loss: Miss Hyde-Whyte 食欲不振と体重減：ハイド＝ホワイトさん	
	Case history 9	Alcohol abuse: Mr Wakefield アルコール乱用：ウェイクフィールド氏	

Unit 8	Elimination 排泄		88
	Case history 10	Urinary incontinence: Mrs Carter コンチネンス・ケア（尿失禁のケア）：カーター夫人	
	Case history 11	Constipation: Mr Norton 便秘：ノートン氏	

Unit 9	Personal care — cleansing and dressing, skin care 日常生活の介護 — 洗浄と身支度, スキンケア		100
	Case history 12	Geriatric deterioration: Mrs McBride 加齢による機能低下：マックブライド夫人	
	Case history 13	Eczema: Mr Dafnis 湿疹：ダフニス氏	

Unit 10	Sleeping 睡眠		112
	Case history 14	Sleep disorder: Mrs Bell 睡眠障害：ベル夫人	

Unit 11	Working and playing 仕事と遊び		122
	Case history 15	After myocardial infarction: Mr Khan 心筋梗塞のその後：カーン氏	
	Case history 16	Diabetic retinopathy: Mrs Hamilton 糖尿病性網膜症：ハミルトン夫人	

Unit 12	Sexuality 性		134
	Case history 17	Erectile dysfunction: Mr Johns 勃起障害：ジョンズ氏	
	Case history 18	Dysmenorrhoea: Mrs Hall 月経困難：ホール夫人	

Unit 13	Anxiety, stress and depression 不安, ストレス, うつ		146
	Case history 19	A panic attack: Mr Reeves パニック発作：リーヴズ氏	
	Case history 20	Worries at school: Mel 学校での心配ごと：メル	

Unit 14	Dementia and confusion 認知症と錯乱状態		160
	Case history 21	A wife whose husband has severe dementia: Mr Georges 認知症の夫を持つ妻：ジョージズ夫人	

Unit 15　Pain　痛み　　　　　　　　　　　　　　　　　　　　　168
　　　Case history 22　Migraine attacks: Miss Carter
　　　　　　　　　　　　偏頭痛発作：カーターさん

Thinking about (reflection) practice: exercise　　　　　　　　　178
実践について考える（振り返り）：問題

II　Glossary of medical and colloquial names　　182
病気の医学名と口語名の用語集

III　Abbreviations used in nursing
看護で使用される略語

Introduction　はじめに　　　　　　　　　　　　　　　　　　　190

Abbreviations　略語　　　　　　　　　　　　　　　　　　　　190

IV　Units of measurement
計量単位

Units of measurement: international system of units (SI),
the metric system and conversions　　　　　　　　　　　　　240
計量単位：国際単位系 (SI)，メートル法と換算

Measurements, equivalents and conversions
(SI or metric and imperial)　　　　　　　　　　　　　　　　248
度量法，等価量，そして換算 (SI 単位，メートル法，そして英国度量衡法)

I COMMUNICATION IN NURSING

Unit 1 INTRODUCTION

Being able to communicate is an essential skill for all health professionals and it is particularly important for nurses who are with people and their families for many hours a day. It is not always easy to understand what people are saying or to get them to understand what you are trying to tell them. Sometimes nurses who qualified in the UK have difficulties understanding people who have regional accents and many patients use different words for feelings and everyday events. Some of these words are part of this chapter, and Chapter 2 (Colloquial English) gives you lots more examples.

Nurses need to communicate so they can find out about the people in their care by taking a nursing history, give them information about their care and teach them about managing their illness.

This chapter will help you with some of the questions needed to take a nursing history and plan care based on a commonly used Activities of Living Model of Nursing (see Roper et al 1996) and some other important nursing issues (e.g. confusion and anxiety). Short case histories that focus on a particular activity are included to help you with some common situations. There are extracts from dialogues (conversations) between nurses and people/clients/relatives that give you examples of what they may say to you in answer to your questions. These case histories will be useful when you deal with similar situations at work, and later reflect on the positive and negative features of a particular conversation you had with a patient/client and their family.

Note: All the people and case histories used are fictitious and are not based on any persons we have nursed or met when supervising students.

I 看護におけるコミュニケーション

Unit 1　　　　　　　　　　　　　　　　　　　　　　　　　　はじめに

　意思の疎通をはかる能力は，すべての医療専門職にとって必須である。1日のうちの長時間を人々とその家族と過ごす看護師にとって，コミュニケーション能力はとりわけ重要である。人々が話していることを理解すること，あるいは，自分が言おうとしていることを相手に理解してもらうことは，必ずしも容易ではない。英国で資格を得ている看護師は，方言で話す人の発音を理解するのが難しいことがある。また，多くの患者は，それぞれに異なる言葉で感情や日々の出来事を表現する。本章ではそうした表現の一部を紹介し，さらに次章(「日常英語表現」〔本対訳書では省略〕)においてより多くの実例を示す。

　看護師は次のような目的でコミュニケーションを取る必要がある。1. 看護歴を取ることによって，看護中の患者について知る，2. 患者の看護について情報を提供する，3. 患者に疾病の管理について指導する。

　本章は，看護歴を取る際，広く用いられている Activities of Living Model of Nursing (Roper ほか 1996 参照) に基づいて看護計画を立てる際に，必要となる質問並びにその他の看護上重要な問題(例：混乱や不安)において読者に役立つだろう。特定の活動に焦点を絞った短い症例を示すことにより，(ある症例における)一般的な状況を理解する手助けとしている。看護師が人々・患者・親族と交わす対話(会話)を引用することにより，あなたの質問に対してこうした人々がどのように答えるかの例を提示している。こうした症例は，あなたが実務で同様の状況を扱うときに有用となるだろう。また，患者やその家族と交わした特定の会話の良かった点と悪かった点について反省する際にも役立つだろう。

注記：本書に扱われている人々並びに症例はみなフィクションであり，私たちがこれまで看護をしてきた人々や学生の指導時に会った実在の人々ではない。

Unit 2   GETTING STARTED

The first words you say to a person are very important — you need to get it right. You need to say who you are and why you are there. What you say will depend on the situation, but you might start with:

> 'Hello [or good morning/good evening] Mrs Jones I am Nurse [your last name/surname/family name].'

or just use your first and last names and say that you are the nurse who will be caring for them for the shift (or whatever is appropriate).

Ask Mrs Jones what she likes to be called. You will hear patients and nurses using lots of different forms of address: for example, the titles Mr, Ms, Miss, Mrs or Dr with the last name, or first names, or sometimes endearments such as love, dear, gran, nan, grandpa, honey, darling, mate, pet, hen, duck, etc. As a general rule it is not acceptable to use endearments when speaking to patients. Do not use a person's first name unless they ask you to do so. It is important to follow a person's wishes about their preferred form of address — make sure that this is written in the nursing notes for all nurses to read.

Once you know what the person wants to be called you can start to get the information needed to plan nursing care, explain the care, tests or treatment planned, and answer any questions. Remember that if you cannot answer a person's question it is important to get another nurse, doctor or other healthcare professional to do so.

Whenever possible ask simple questions that will ensure you get the exact information needed, and avoid using jargon. For example, saying to Mrs Jones 'I will be back to do your vital signs or obs[1]' will mean nothing to her — you will need to explain that you will be back to record her blood pressure, temperature, pulse and respiration. Always check any prepared documents that arrive from the admissions office or the emergency department the person's details may have changed or there might be a mistake.

---

1. obs observation または observation の略。バイタル・サインと同様の意味で使われる。

Unit 2　　　　　　　　　　　　　　　　　　　　会話の開始

　最初の一言は大変重要である。正しいスタートを切らなければならない。自分がだれで，なぜそこにいるのかを，伝える必要がある。何を言うかは状況によるが，次のように始めることができるだろう。

> **「こんにちは（おはようございます / こんばんは），ジョーンズさん。私は看護師の～（名字）です。」**

　あるいは，名字と名前，そしてこれから患者のケアを担当すると（あるいは何であれ適切なことを）言う。

　ジョーンズさんに自分が何と呼ばれたいか，尋ねるとよい。患者も看護師も実にさまざまな呼びかけ方をする。例えば，ミスター，ミセス，ミズ，ドクターといった敬称に名字をつけたもの，あるいは名前，ときには親愛を表す表現，例えばラブ，ディア，グラン〔gran「おばあちゃん」〕，ナン〔nan「おばあちゃん」〕，グランパ〔grandpa「おじいちゃん」〕，ハニー，ダーリン，メイト〔mate「友達」〕，ペット〔pet「いい子」〕，ヘン〔hen「お嬢さん」〕，ダック〔duck「かわいい人」〕，などである。一般的に，患者に対して親愛の呼びかけ表現を使うのは好ましくない。ファーストネームで呼ぶのは，患者がそうしてほしいと言ったときだけである。呼び名について患者の希望を取り入れることは大切である。この呼称は，すべての看護師が読めるよう看護記録に確実に書いておくとよい。

　相手が希望する呼び名がわかったら，看護計画の立案，看護・検査・治療計画の説明に必要な情報収集を開始し，質問にも答え始めることができる。もし患者の質問に答えることができなければ，ほかの看護師・医師・その他の医療専門職に対応してもらうことが重要である。

　常にできるだけ単純な質問をして，必要とする正確な情報を得られるようにする。そして，専門用語を使うのを避ける。例えば，ジョーンズ夫人に「バイタル・サインあるいは obs のチェックをするために戻ります。」と言っても通じないだろう。血圧，体温，脈拍，呼吸の記録をするために戻るのだということを説明する必要がある。入院手続きや救急科から届いた書類はいつも確認をすること。患者の詳細についての記載に変更が生じていたり，間違いがありうるからである。

Biographical data

—You will need to start with the assessment sheet, finding out details about your patient such as their full name, where they live (address) and who with.

'Mrs Jones can you tell me your full name [first name or forename followed by last name which is also called the surname or family name] and your address and telephone number.'

If you ask where they live patients might say 'In the town' or 'With my husband', so it is best to ask for the address (house number/name, the street, the town, county and the postcode[2]). If you have problems spelling a name or address, always ask the patient or their relative to spell it out letter by letter or even copy it out for you — it must be accurate. It is important to ask your patient's age and date of birth, e.g. 57 years, 22/2/1946. In the UK dates are always written in the order day, month and year.

—Always ask the name and address of the patient's next of kin, and get telephone numbers (daytime and for use at night) in case it is necessary to contact family members. Obviously this might be necessary if the patient's condition worsens, but it might be to say that the person can come home so please can the family bring in outdoor clothes. If the next of kin lives many miles away the patient may give you contact details of a friend or neighbour (someone living close to them).

—An assessment includes asking about the patient's religion (if any) or spiritual needs, so you can plan care that ensures any religious, spiritual or cultural needs are met. These needs may include attending a religious service/ceremony, having a visit from a religious leader, priest, minister, mullah, rabbi, etc., or having facilities for prayer, needing to fast or having special food.

---

2. postcode 英国では、住所に番号・番地がなく Rose Cottage や Stone House といった家の名前のみの場合がある。

経歴

―まずアセスメント・シートを用いて，フルネームや住所・同居者などといった患者についての詳細を知ることから始める必要がある。

> 「ジョーンズさん，あなたの氏名（名前「ファースト・ネーム」または「フォアネーム」，と苗字「ラストネーム」，「サーネーム」，または「ファミリー・ネーム」とも言う）それから住所と電話番号を教えてください。」

もし「どこに住んでいますか」と尋ねると，患者は「町に」とか「夫と一緒に」などと答えるかもしれない。したがって，もっともよいのは，住所（家の番号／名前，通り，町，郡，郵便番号など）を尋ねることである。名前や住所のつづりがはっきりしない場合は，患者または親族に一字一字つづりを言ってもらったり，書いてもらったりすること―つづりは正確でなければならない。もう１つ重要なのは，患者の年齢と生年月日を聞くことである。例えば，57 歳，22 日 2 月 1946 年というように。英国では常に日，月，年の順番で書く。（例：22/2/1946）

―いつも患者の〔最〕近親者の名前と住所を聞くこと。また家族に連絡が必要な場合に備えて，電話番号（日中につながるものと夜間につながるもの）も聞いておく。これは患者の容態が悪くなったときには明らかに必要になるだろうし，患者が退院できるので外出着を持ってきてほしいと頼む場合もありえる。近親者が遠くに住んでいる場合は，患者は友人や隣人（近くに住む人）の連絡先を伝えることもある。

―アセスメントには，（もしあれば）患者の宗教や精神的欲求について尋ねることが含まれる。そうすることで，患者の宗教的，精神的，文化的欲求を満たせるような看護計画を立案することができる。こうした欲求としては，宗教的礼拝／儀式への出席，宗教的指導者・司祭・牧師〔特にプロテスタント教会における〕・マラ〔イスラム教指導者〕・ラビ〔ユダヤ教の聖職者〕などの訪問を受けること，祈祷場所の確保，断食の必要性，特別な食事の提供などがある。

'What religion are you Mrs Jones?'

Then you can ask appropriate questions, such as

'Will you want to see your minister or visit the hospital chapel?'

In the UK many patients will answer with the abbreviation for their religion, e.g. 'C of E' for Church of England or 'RC' for Roman Catholic.

Work (employment) history

You will need to ask the patient if they work. This usually means paid work, but many people in the UK do unpaid voluntary work and this should also be recorded on the assessment form.

Once you know that the patient works you can get more details. The type of work may be influencing their health (e.g. exposure to substances such as asbestos that can cause cancer, work in a dusty environment and chest diseases, or back pain where heavy objects must be moved). The length of time off work following an operation will depend on the type of work the patient does, and in some situations patients cannot go back to their old job (e.g. some driving jobs following a heart attack (myocardial infarction)).

The question:

'What do you do?'

usually means 'What is your work?.' Patients may tell you where they work (i.e. the company name) rather than the type of job they do. So if they say

'I've been at Clarks since I left school and that's nearly 30 years.'

you will have to ask:

'What job do you do at Clarks?'

「ジョーンズさん，あなたの宗教は何ですか？」

それから適切な質問へと進める。例えば，

「牧師に会いたいですか，病院内の礼拝堂に行きたいですか？」など。

英国では多くの患者が自分の宗教を略語で答えるだろう。例えば，英国教会はC of E (Church of England)，ローマカトリックはRC (Roman Catholic) と。

職歴（雇用歴）

患者が働いているかどうか尋ねる必要がある。通常，有給の仕事を意味するが，英国では多くの人が無給のボランティアの仕事をしている。無給の仕事もアセスメント記録に記載されるべきである。

患者が働いていることがわかったら，さらに詳しいことを聞くことができる。仕事の種類は患者の健康に影響を与える場合がある（例えば，アスベストのようにがんを引き起こす物質との接触，ほこりっぽい環境での仕事と胸部疾患，重い物を動かすところでの腰痛）。手術後仕事を再開できるまでの期間は，患者の仕事の種類による。場合によっては，患者は元の仕事に戻れないこともある（例えば，心臓発作《心筋梗塞》後の車を運転する仕事など）。

質問：

「あなたは何をしていらっしゃいますか？」

通常これは「あなたの仕事は何ですか？」を意味する。患者は，どのような仕事をしているかではなく，どこで働いているか（すなわち会社名）を答えることがある。

「学校を出てからクラークスに勤めていて，30年近くになります。」

患者がこのように答えた場合は，次のように尋ねる必要がある。

「クラークスではどんな仕事をしていますか？」

'Do you work full time or part time?'
'How many hours do you work in a week?'
'Do you work shifts?'
(This relates to irregular hours, e.g. in a hospital or factory.)
'How long have you been doing this job?'
'Do you have a stressful job? Do you work late or have to take work home?'

If patients are not working you need to find out why - are they retired from work and, if so, ask what type of work they used to do, looking after children or a relative, looking for work, studying or unable to work for health reasons.

Reason for admission or contact with health services and medical details

—*The patient's understanding of reason for admission/treatment, etc.* It is important to find out exactly why the patient thinks they have visited the general practitioner/practice nurse[3], or come into hospital or the care home. It might be correct to ask a direct question such as:

'What do you think is the matter with you?'

or

'Tell me why you have come in today.'

This last type of comment might be used for a patient coming in for a planned operation. The patient may say something like

'I've come in to get my cataract done [operated on].'

---

3. practice nurse「開業看護師」英国では国が運営するNHS〔National Health Service: 国民保健サービス〕により全国民に健康医療サービスが行われる。英国の多くの就業看護師はこのNHSに雇用されており、それに対し、自身で開業、または開業医に雇われている看護師を practice nurse と呼ぶ。また、英国では日本の看護師にくらべ業務内容が広範にわたる。

「常勤ですか，パートですか？」
「1週間の労働時間はどれくらいですか？」
「交替制で仕事をしますか？」
　（交替制があると不規則な勤務時間となる，例えば，病院や工場など）
「今の仕事をどれくらい長く続けていますか？」
「ストレスの多い仕事ですか。残業したり，家に仕事を持ち帰らなければなりませんか？」

　患者が仕事をしていない場合は，その理由を知る必要がある。退職したのであれば，以前はどのような仕事をしていたのか尋ねること。子供や親族の世話をしているのか，求職中か，勉強をしているのか，健康上の理由で働くことができないのか，などの質問をする。

入院または医療を受ける理由と詳しい医療情報

―患者が入院・治療などの理由をどのように理解しているか。大事なのは，一般開業医や開業看護師を受診した理由，病院や介護施設に来た理由を患者自身がどう考えているかを正確に知ることである。直接的な質問をするのもよいだろう。例えば，

「何が問題だとお考えですか？」

あるいは

「なぜ今日ここにいらしたのか話してください。」

この質問は，手術に来院した患者に適用されるだろう。患者は次のように答えるかもしれない。

「白内障をやってもらう［手術をしてもらう］ために来ました。」

Sometimes you will need to use questions such as:

> 'Have you been having some problems at home?'

and the patient may say:

> 'I've been having dizzy turns [vertigo] when I keel over [fall over].'

or

> 'I had a spell [a period of time] of feeling very down [depressed mood] but that has cleared up [got better, disappeared] now.'

You will also need to check that the family know why the patient has been admitted.

—*Past medical history and family history.* You will need to ask about past illnesses or operations. For example, a patient coming in for a routine operation may have type 1 diabetes or they may have severe arthritis that makes walking very difficult and you will need to plan care accordingly. You might ask:

> 'Have you ever had any serious illnesses in the past?'
> 'Have you ever had an operation?'
> 'Have you ever been in hospital before?'
> 'Have you ever had any accidents or injuries?'
> 'Is there anything else you'd like to tell me?'

As some illnesses, such as some types of heart disease and diabetes, may run in certain families (familial) you will also need to ask about the family medical history:

> 'Are there any serious illnesses in your family?'

—*Allergies.* Always ask about any allergies, including foods, drugs (see below) and other substances such as washing powders:

> 'Are you allergic to anything?'
> 'Have you any allergies?'

次のような質問の仕方をしなければならないこともある。

「家で何か問題がありましたか？」

患者は次のように答えるかもしれない。

「ふらふらして倒れる［転倒する］ときにはいつも目が回っていました［めまいがしました］」。

あるいは

「私はひととき［一時期］すごく気分が落ち込んだことがありました［憂うつな気分だった］が，今はよくなり［回復し，〔憂うつな気分は〕なくなり］ました。」

また，患者の家族が入院理由を知っているかどうかをチェックする必要がある。

――*既往歴と家族歴*。過去の病気や手術について尋ねる必要がある。例えば，日常的な手術を受けに来た患者にⅠ型糖尿病があったり，歩くのが困難な重い関節炎があったりするので，それぞれの患者に合った看護計画を立てる必要があるだろう。次のような質問をすることができる。

「これまでに重い病気にかかったことはありますか？」
「手術を受けたことはありますか？」
「以前入院したことはありますか？」
「事故にあったり，怪我をしたことはありますか？」
「何かほかに伝えておきたいことはありますか？」

ある種の心臓病や糖尿病のように，病気によっては一族に遺伝（家族性）なので，家族の病歴についても尋ねる必要がある。

「ご家族に重い病気の方はいますか？」

――*アレルギー*。常にあらゆるアレルギーについて尋ねること。例えば，食物，薬剤（下記を参照），洗剤やそのほかの物質など。

「何かにアレルギーがありますか？」
「アレルギーがありますか？」

It might be necessary to ask the family, for example, if the patient is a child, has dementia or is unconscious.

—*Drugs.* It is necessary to ask all patients/clients if they are taking any drugs, but it is worth remembering that some patients will associate the word 'drugs' with illegal substances and drug misuse, so you can ask:

> 'Are you taking any medicines (or drugs)?'

Always ask patients about all types of drugs, including those prescribed by a doctor or nurse, drugs they buy at the chemist (pharmacy) or supermarket (over-the-counter drugs), natural remedies such as St. John's Wort, and if appropriate ask about recreational (illegal) drugs[4] such as cannabis. It is vital to know about any drug allergies (e.g. penicillin) or adverse drug reactions. Always ask and make sure that this is recorded in all the relevant nursing documentation.

Physical function and effects of current illness on daily living or work

Many areas of physical function, such as mobility (moving about), are covered in the dialogue section (see pp. 28-178), but you will need to ask how the current illness affects everyday life.
For example:

> 'Is there anything you need help with at home, such as getting out of bed or making a cup of tea?'
> 'How often does your neighbour come in to help you?'
> 'Are you still able to work?'

---

4. recreational drugs「レクリエーショナル・ドラッグ」治療用ではなく快楽追求のための麻薬。

患者が小児の場合，あるいは認知症を患っていたり，意識がないといった場合には，家族に問診する必要があるかもしれない。

——薬物。すべての患者/クライエントに現在薬物を飲んでいるかどうか尋ねる必要がある。患者によっては，drugs「薬物」という言葉を違法物質や薬物乱用に結びつける可能性があることを覚えておくとよい。したがって，次のように尋ねることができる。

「何か薬(または薬物)を飲んでいますか？」

患者にはあらゆる種類の薬剤について尋ねること。医師や看護師が処方したものから，薬剤師のところ（薬局）やスーパー（市販薬）で購入したもの，セント・ジョーンズ・ワートのような生薬，そして必要なら，大麻のようなレクリエーショナル・ドラッグ（違法）麻薬についても尋ねる。非常に重要なのは，薬物アレルギー（例：ペニシリン）や薬剤による副作用について知ることである。常にこうしたことについて尋ね，関連するすべての看護記録に残るようにすること。

身体機能と現在の病気による日常生活や仕事への影響

さまざまな領域の身体機能，例えば運動能力（動き回れること）などは，会話のセクション（原文 26 〜 178 頁参照）で扱われている。しかし，現在の病気がどのように日常生活に影響を与えているか尋ねる必要があるだろう。
例えば，

「家庭で手助けが必要なことはありますか，例えばベッドから出たり，お茶を入れたりするということで」
「近所の人はあなたの手助けにどのくらいの頻度で来てくれますか？」
「あなたは今も仕事ができますか？」

Social history

—*Support networks* are important particularly after discharge. You can ask questions that include:

'Do your family live close by?'
'Who will be at home to look after you when you are discharged?'
'Will you be able to stay with your family until you are able to manage back at home?'

—*Type of home.* Although you know the patient's address, you also need to know about the type of home they have. Patients who live alone in a big house may be unable to keep it heated or clean after discharge, and a patient who lives in a flat up several fights of stairs may need to be found a ground-floor flat before they can go home. You will need to ask questions that include:

'Do you live in a house, bungalow, flat, bedsit, etc.?'

(A bedsit is a room used for both sleeping and daytime activities with the use of shared kitchen and bathroom.)

'How do you heat your home?'

(Patients may not be able to manage an open fire or may not use expensive heating if they are living on a low wage, pension or benefits.)

'Do you have good neighbours?'

(The patient may be relying on the neighbours to check the house, feed pets, take in post and do things like cutting the grass while they are in hospital.)

—*Social problems due to present condition/admission.* Patients admitted as an emergency may be worried about children or others such as older relatives at home who depend on them. Many people in the UK have pet animals such as a cat or dog and you should always ask if

社会歴

—支援ネットワークは重要で，とりわけ退院後に重要になる。次のような質問をすることができる。

> 「ご家族は近くに住んでいますか？」
> 「退院したらだれが家で世話をしてくれますか？」
> 「家に帰って自分でどうにかやれるようになるまで，家族のところにいることはできますか？」

—*住居の種類*。住所だけでなく，どのような種類の住居なのか知る必要がある。大きな家に1人で住んでいる患者は，退院後，家を暖かい温度に保ったり，きれいに維持することができないかもしれない。また，アパートの上のほうの階に住んでいる患者は，家に戻る前に1階のアパートを見つけなければならないかもしれない。次のように質問する必要があるだろう。

> 「住まいは一戸建て，平屋，アパート，それともワンルームのアパートですか？」

(bedsit「ワンルームのアパート」は，台所と風呂場は共用で，1部屋を寝室としても日中の活動の場としても使う部屋である。)

> 「家はどうやって暖めますか？」

(患者は暖炉の火を扱えないかもしれない。また，低賃金，年金，生活保護で暮らしている場合，お金のかかる暖房を使えないかもしれない。)

> 「近所の方は親切ですか？」

(患者は，入院中に，家の様子を見てもらったり，ペットのえさやり，郵便物の受け取り，草刈りなどといったことを近所の人にお願いしているかもしれない。)

—*現在の病気／入院による社会生活上の問題*。緊急入院した患者は，子供や家にいる高齢の親族といった扶養家族について心配をするかもしれない。英国では

they have a pet, and if someone is caring for them.

'Do you have any pets at home?'
'What's your cat's name?'
'Who is feeding Harry?'

You will need to listen very carefully, as a patient with dementia, for example, may keep repeating the name of the pet animal rather than tell you the details. Patients can be very anxious about the care of their pet animals while they are in hospital or a care home.

—*Hobbies and interests.*

'How do you spend your free time?'
'How much exercise do you take?'
'Do you play any sports?'
'Have you any hobbies?'
'Do you like to watch TV [television] or listen to music?'

—*Contacts with and input from other health and social care professionals.*
Many older patients will already be in contact with a wide range of health and social care professions, such as a district nurse[5], health visitor[6], practice nurse, general practitioner (family doctor), physiotherapist, occupational therapist, speech and language therapist, dietician, podiatrist[7] or social worker. You should ask about this and find out who comes, how often and what they do:

'Do you see the nurse at home?'
'What do the nurses do?'
'Do they come in everyday?'

---

5. **district nurse**「地区看護師」担当地域の住宅治療中の患者に訪問看護を行う。
6. **health visitor**「訪問保健師」担当地域の住民を訪問して健康管理や病気予防などについて指導を行う。
7. **podiatrist**「足病専門医」足の病気を専門に治療する医師。英国では chiropodists と呼ばれていたこともある。

多くの人が猫や犬などのペットを飼っている。患者がペットを飼っているかどうか，留守中に世話をする人がいるのかどうか，についても尋ねるべきである。

　　「家にペットがいますか？」
　　「あなたの猫の名前は何ですか？」
　　「今だれがハリーにえさをあげていますか？」

このことはとても注意深く聞く必要がある。なぜなら，認知症などの患者は，詳しい説明をするのではなく，ペットの名前を繰り返し言い続けたりすることがあるからだ。患者は，病院に入院中または介護施設に入所中は，自分のペットの世話についてとても心配することがある。

―*趣味と興味*。

　　「暇なときは何をしていますか？」
　　「運動はどのくらいしますか？」
　　「何かスポーツをしますか？」
　　「趣味はありますか？」
　　「TV［テレビ］を見たり音楽を聴いたりするのは好きですか。」

―*ほかの医療専門職や社会的介護の専門職とのつながりや，そうした人たちからの情報の入手*。高齢の患者の多くは，すでに幅広い医療並びに社会的介護の専門職と接触している可能性がある。例えば，地区看護師，訪問保健師，開業看護師，一般開業医（家庭医），理学療法士，作業療法士，言語療法士，栄養士，足病専門医，ソーシャル・ワーカーなどである。このことについて尋ね，だれが，どのくらいの頻度で来て，何をしているか知る必要がある。

　　「家で看護師に診てもらっていますか？」
　　「看護師は何をしますか？」
　　「毎日来ますか？」

Lifestyle

During the nursing assessment you will need to find out about lifestyle or behaviour that can influence health in both good or bad ways (e.g. the type of foods eaten, amount of exercise, alcohol intake, use of drugs, use of tobacco, sexual behaviour and high-risk leisure activities). Often a person's lifestyle or behaviour is sensitive and they may feel embarrassed or guilty if you ask lots of questions. Thus direct questioning does not always work well in this situation, but often you will be able to get the information as the patient talks about their lifestyle and view of health. For example, a patient may tell you, without any prompting, that they know they do not get enough exercise and you can find out more by asking them what they mean. Sometimes, however, you will need to ask more directly and the sort of questions that may be needed to get information about some of these lifestyle issues are discussed in the following section under the related activity.

生活習慣

　看護アセスメントを行う間，患者の健康に良い影響あるいは悪い影響を与える生活習慣や行動について聞き出す必要がある（例えば，食べている食物の種類，運動量，アルコールの摂取量，薬の使用，喫煙，性行動，危険を伴う余暇活動）。人の生活習慣や行動は扱いが難しい話題で，たくさんの質問をすると患者は困惑したり後ろめたい気分になるかもしれない。従って，この場合，直接的な質問をするのが常にうまくいくとは限らない。むしろ，患者が自分の生活習慣や健康観について話をしているときに情報を得られることがよくある。例えば，患者は，人に促されなくても，自分は運動を十分にしていないのがわかっているとあなたに語ることもある。それが何を意味するか尋ねることで，より多くのことを知ることができるだろう。しかしながら，ときには，より直截に質問する必要がある。そしてそのような，直接的に尋ねる必要のある，生活習慣における問題点のいくつかに関する質問は，次のセクションで関連する活動別に説明していく。

Unit 3　BREATHING

Some nursing/medical or Standard English words and corresponding colloquial words and expressions associated with breathing are given in Box. 1.

Note: Colloquial expressions used in the case histories[8] and example conversations are explained in brackets [...].

BOX. 1

Words associated with breathing

Nursing/medical or Standard English words	Colloquial (everyday) or slang (very informal) words and expressions used by patients
Dyspnoea	Breathlessness; out of breath; puffed; short of breath; fighting for breath (severe cases)
Expectorate	To bring up/cough up phlegm; spit
Expiration	Breathing out
Inhaler for drugs	Puffer
Inspiration	Breathing in
Respiration	Breathing
Sputum	Phlegm (pronounced flem)

Case history 1　　Dyspnoea: Mr and Mrs Ryan

Mr Ryan has been admitted to the medical assessment unit[9] with a chest infection causing an exacerbation [worsening] of his chronic obstructive pulmonary disease (COPD). He is very distressed and finding it hard to breathe. His wife tells you that 'His breathing has been bad for years
5　and he can't get about much these days' — meaning that his mobility

---

8. **case histories** この注記における case histories は、各 case history（症例）の前書き部分に記された個々の患者の病歴の説明を指していると考えられる。
9. **medical assessment unit** 「メディカル・アセスメント病棟」救急や GP（かかりつけ医）の紹介で訪れた患者を検査・治療し、必要があればさらに専門病棟に患者を送る。

Unit 3　　　　　　　　　　　　　　　　　　　　　　　　　　呼吸

呼吸に関連する看護・医学用語あるいは標準英語，対応する口語的な用語と表現を Box. 1 にまとめた。

注記：病歴と会話例文中における口語的な表現には，〔　〕内に説明を加えた。

Box. 1

呼吸に関連する用語

看護 / 医学用語， または標準英語の用語	患者が使う口語的（日常的） または，俗語（非常にくだけた）用語と表現
呼吸困難	息切れ；息を切らした；息を切らした；息を切らす；息をするのが苦しい（重い場合）
〔痰を〕喀出する	痰を出す / 咳で痰が出る；〔痰を〕吐く
呼気	息を吐くこと
薬の吸入器	吸入器
吸気	息を吸うこと
呼吸	呼吸
痰	痰（発音は [flem]）

症例 1　　呼吸困難：ライアン氏とライアン夫人

ライアン氏は，肺感染症により慢性閉塞性肺疾患（COPD）が増悪〔悪化〕してきており，メディカル・アセスメント病棟に入院している。彼は大変苦しんでおり，呼吸が困難である。彼の妻は，「彼は何年間も呼吸の具合が悪く，最近はあまり歩き回れない ─ 運動能力が低下している」と言っている。ライアン夫人か

is reduced. You can get the biographical data from Mrs Ryan, and as soon as Mr Ryan's condition improves you can find out more about his breathing and related problems. You might also want to ask Mrs Ryan if her husband becomes confused or mixed up [disorientated], as this may be a sign of reduced oxygen getting to the brain (caused by hypoxia), or if he is more drowsy [sleepy] than normal. This may happen if there is too much carbon dioxide in the arterial blood (hypercapnia).

2

Nurse: Mrs Ryan have you noticed a change in your husband's mental state recently, does he get confused?
Mrs R.: Now you come to mention it he does seem a bit dotty [silly] sometimes. You know, not always knowing where he is.
Nurse: Hello Mr Ryan tell me about the problems you have with your breathing.
Mr R.: I'm breathless most of the time but the infection made it much worse — I was really frightened and felt that I was fighting for breath until the treatment (more bronchodilators, corticosteroids[10] and antibiotic therapy) started to work [became effective].
Nurse: Before the infection how was your breathing? Were you breathless sitting still?
Mr R.: Oh no, only when I tried to walk about.
Nurse: Can you normally get upstairs in one go [without stopping]?
Mr R.: Only if I rest on the landing [flat part of a staircase] and get my breath back [recover].
Nurse: How far can you walk on the level without getting breathless?
Mr R.: I can get as far as the back garden but I'm fair jiggered [exhausted, breathless] after.

10.corticosteroid「コルチコステロイド剤, 副腎皮質ステロイド」コレステロールの側鎖切断により生成するプレグネノロンを出発点として副腎皮質において産生・分泌されるステロイド・ホルモンの総称 = corticoid。略語 CS。

らは生活史データを聴取でき，ライアン氏の病状が改善し次第，彼の呼吸状態やそれに関連する諸問題について〔本人から〕より多くのことを知ることができるだろう。ライアン氏が困惑したり混乱したり［見当識障害］している場合，（低酸素症により）脳に送られる酸素が減少している兆候かもしれないので，この点についても尋ねるべきである。また，彼が通常よりも眠い［眠気がある］かについても質問するとよい。動脈血中に二酸化炭素が過剰にある（高炭酸ガス血症）とそのように感じることがある。

看護師： ライアンさん，近頃ご主人の精神状態の変化で気づいたことはありますか？ご主人は混乱しますか？

R婦人： 今そう言われてみると，主人はときどきちょっとおかしな［ぼんやりした］状態のときが確かにあります。そう，ときどき自分がどこにいるのかわからないのです。

看護師： こんにちは，ライアンさん。呼吸で困っていることを聞かせてください。

R氏： ほとんど常に息切れがしているのですが，感染症のせいでもっと悪くなりました ― 本当に恐ろしかったです。治療（追加の気管支拡張剤，コルチコステロイド剤，抗生物質による治療）が効き始めるまでは息をしようと必死でした。

看護師： 感染症にかかる前は呼吸はどうでしたか？じっと座っていても息切れがしましたか？

R氏： いいえ，歩き回ろうとしたときだけです。

看護師： 通常，一気に［止まらずに］階段を上ることはできますか？

R氏： 踊り場［階段の平らな部分］で息をつかないと［回復しないと］上れません。

看護師： 平らな所は息切れせずにどのくらい歩けますか？

R氏： 裏庭ぐらいまでは行けますが，その後はへとへとになります［疲れ果てます，息切れがします］。

Nurse: Is there anything else about your breathing? Do you wheeze [make an audible noise when breathing]?

Mr R.: Yes, I do wheeze and my chest often feels tight, but Dr Singh is going to put me on something new [prescribe a different drug], so hopefully that will do the trick [hopes the new treatment will be effective] — fingers crossed [hope for good luck].

Nurse: Hope so. What medicines were you taking at home before you came into the ward?

Mr R.: The blue inhaler [salbutamol inhaler], and the antibiotics from the GP[11] for the infection.

Nurse: Are you using oxygen at home?

Mr R.: Yes, for up to 15 hours a day. It's OK, we have a machine that takes some gases out of the air and leaves the oxygen [oxygen concentrator] for me, so the missus [wife] doesn't need to keep changing cylinders and I can get around in the house and out as far as the back garden.

Nurse: What else helps your breathing?

Mr R.: Well — sitting up and leaning on the table helps, but when I'm very chesty [trouble with chest, coughing] it's better to sleep downstairs in an armchair. At least the wife gets some sleep even if I don't. A while ago I started doing relaxation exercises and that helps when I feel panicky [frightened], but they didn't work last night — worse luck.

Nurse: Do you still smoke?

Mr R.: No, not for years.

Nurse: When did you stop smoking?

Mr R.: I used to smoke roll-ups [cigarettes that the patient makes himself] and I cut myself down [reduced the number of

---

11. GP「かかりつけ医」英国では、患者はまず登録してある GP (General Practitioner) にかかり、そこで専門医にかかる必要があるかどうか判断される。国営のため、多くの場合は自己負担額が低額だが、待ち時間の長さから高額の料金を払ってプライベートの医療機関を利用する患者も少なくない。

看護師： 呼吸についてほかに何かありますか。息をするとぜーぜーしますか〔呼吸するときに雑音が聞こえますか〕？

R氏： はい。ぜーぜーいいますし，よく胸が締めつけられる感じがします。でも，シン先生が何か新しい薬を出して〔これまでと違う薬を処方して〕くださるので，それが効く〔新しい治療が効果を出す〕ことを願います。─〔人差し指の上に中指を重ねて〕効きますように〔幸運を祈る〕。

看護師： そうだといいですね。入院する前は家でどんな薬を飲んでいましたか？

R氏： 青い吸入薬〔サルブタモール吸入薬〕と，GP〔かかりつけの先生〕が感染症用に出してくれた抗生物質です。

看護師： 家では酸素を使っていますか？

R氏： はい，1日15時間以内で使っています。問題はありませんよ。家に機械があって，空気中から気体〔窒素〕を取り除いて，酸素を残してくれるんです〔酸素濃縮器〕。かみさん〔妻〕はシリンダーをしょっちゅう換える必要はないし，家の中を歩き回れるし，裏庭までなら外にも行けますよ。

看護師： ほかに呼吸の助けになるものはありますか。

R氏： えーと，椅子に座って，テーブルに寄りかかるのが役に立ちます。でも，すごく胸がおかしい〔胸の具合が悪い，咳が出る〕ときは，階下のひじ掛け椅子で眠る方がいいです。私がだめでも，少なくとも家内は眠れますから。少し前に，リラクゼーションのための訓練を始めまして，パニック状態に陥りそうな〔自暴自棄になりそうな〕ときにはそれが役に立ちます。でも，ゆうべは役に立ちませんでした ─ 運の悪いことに。

看護師： 今もタバコを吸いますか？

R氏： いいえ，何年も吸ってません。

看護師： いつタバコを止めましたか？

R氏： 以前は手巻きタバコ〔患者自身が作る紙巻タバコ〕を吸っていましたが，1日10本まで落としました〔タバコの本数を減らした〕。それから，

50		cigarettes] to 10 a day, and then I said 'That's it. No more' and I haven't smoked for 5 years. It was hard but I was determined to stick to [keep to] no smoking.
	Nurse:	That's good, but do you still cough?
55	Mr R.:	Yes, cough and bring up stuff [phlegm or sputum]. I had a smokers' cough[12] [early morning cough] when I was in the Army, but now I cough any time of the day or night.
	Nurse:	What colour is the sputum you cough up? Has the amount increased?
60	Mr R.:	Really green because of the infection, and much more, and my mouth tastes foul.
65	Nurse:	We sent a specimen to the laboratory earlier, so I'll get you some sputum pots and tissues and some mouthwash. The physiotherapist is on his way up to see you, so he will help you to cough and clear your chest. Do you have any pain with the cough?
	Mr R.:	Not at the moment.
	Nurse:	What about washing and dressing — are you able to manage or do you need some help?
70	Mr R.:	Just need some help to wash my back and feet. She does it at home [meaning Mrs Ryan helps].
	Nurse:	How is your appetite? What about eating and drinking?
	Mr R.:	I'm trying to have a drink every hour like you said, but I can't face [manage] a big meal.
75	Nurse:	I will ask the dietician to visit and discuss it with you, but for today I can give you some nourishing drinks and order snacks or light meals for you.
	Mr R.:	Thanks, that sounds spot on [exactly right].
	Nurse:	Your bed is close to the bathroom and lavatory. Will you be able to walk or will a wheelchair be easier?

---

12. smokers' cough 「喫煙者特有の咳」多くはヘビースモーカーが経験する咳き込みの症状を指す。主に寝起き、早朝に咳が連続して出るため early morning cough とも呼ばれる。

「これでおしまい。もう吸うのはやめだ。」と言って，それ以来 5 年吸ってませんね。大変でしたが，禁煙を守る〔続ける〕決心をしました。

看護師： それはいいことです。でも，まだ咳が出ますか？

R 氏： ええ。咳も，たん〔痰〕も出ます。陸軍にいたときは喫煙者特有の咳〔早朝の咳〕をしていました。でも今は，昼も夜も，いつでも咳が出ます。

看護師： 咳で出るのはどんな色の痰ですか？量は増えましたか？

R 氏： 感染症のせいですごく緑色で，量もだいぶ増えました。口の中がとても気持ち悪いです。

看護師： 先ほど，検体を検査室に送りました。痰つぼとティシュ，口内洗浄液を持ってきましょう。これから理学療法士が来て，うまく咳を出して胸をすっきりさせる方法を教えてくれます。咳をすると痛みますか？

R 氏： 今のところは〔痛みは〕ありません。

看護師： 体を洗うことや，着替えはどうですか ― ご自分でできますか，それとも介助が必要ですか？

R 氏： 背中と足は洗うのをちょっと手伝ってもらっています。家では彼女がやってくれます〔ライアン夫人が手伝っていることを意味している〕。

看護師： 食欲はどうですか？食べたり飲んだりは？

R 氏： 看護師さんに言われたように，1 時間ごとに水分を取るようにしています。でも，量の多い食事はだめです〔食べられません〕。

看護師： 栄養士が来て，話し合えるよう手配します。今日のところは，栄養価の高い飲み物を飲んでください。そしてスナックか軽食を注文しましょう。

R 氏： ありがとう。ちょうどいいです〔まさにぴったりです〕。

看護師： あなたのベッドはトイレ付の浴室と洗面所に近いところにあります。歩いて行けそうですか，それとも車椅子の方がいいですか？

80	Mr R.:	It's not far — I can get there, but after washing I might need some help back.
	Nurse:	How are you sleeping?
	Mr R.:	Don't worry I'll sleep OK tonight — after today with having to call the ambulance and everything I'm knackered [exhausted].
85	Nurse:	Is there anything you would like to ask me?
	Mr R.:	No thanks. You and the doctor explained what was going on [happening] earlier and I do understand about COPD. An 'expert patient[13]' you might say.
	Nurse:	Just ring the bell if you need me. I think Mrs Ryan went to phone your son and have a cup of tea while we did the paperwork. I'll bring her in to you when she gets back.
90		

Other questions

Mr Ryan will find it difficult to talk for long if he is breathless, so you may need to ask some other questions later. Sometimes it will not be necessary to ask because Mr Ryan may tell you extra things as you are attending to his care or he may tell other health professionals, such as the physiotherapist.

Other questions may include some of the following:

> 'Do you have pain or chest discomfort on breathing or coughing?'
> 'Do your ankles get swollen?'
> 'Is there anything that makes you cough worse, such as a smoky or dusty atmosphere, or changes in temperature like going out into the cold? Does any position make it worse?'
> 'Have you noticed any blood in your sputum? Is there a lot of blood or is it streaked with blood?

---

13. expert patient「熟練患者」expert patient の概念は英国で創出され, 慢性疾患の熟練患者 (expert patient) がほかの同じ症状を患う患者を指導・教育することを目的とする, 慢性疾患におけるケア・モデルのひとつ。

R氏：	遠くはないですね — 自分で行けます。でも体を洗った後は戻って来るのに介助が必要がかもしれません。
看護師：	睡眠はどうですか？
R氏：	ご心配なく。今晩はちゃんと眠れると思います。今日は救急車を呼んだり，いろいろあってくたくたです［疲れ切っています］から。
看護師：	何か質問はありますか。
R氏：	いいえ，ありません。看護師さんとドクターが，何があった［起こった］のか説明してくださったし，COPD（慢性閉塞性肺疾患）についてはよく分かっています。「熟練患者」と呼んでいただいてもけっこうですよ。
看護師：	何か用があればベルを鳴らしてください。私たちが書類を書いている間に，奥さんは息子さんに電話をかけたり，お茶を飲んだりしているようです。戻られたらここにお連れしましょう。

その他の質問

ライアン氏は，息切れがするのであれば長く話すのは困難であろう。その他の質問は後ほど尋ねる必要があるかもしれない。場合によっては，質問は必要なくなる。というのも，ライアン氏は，看護を受けている間に，あなたにいろいろなことを話すかもしれない。また，理学療法士など，ほかの医療専門職に話すこともあるだろう。

その他の質問として，次のようなものがあげられる：

「息をしたり咳をするときに，痛みまたは胸部の不快感を伴いますか？」
「くるぶしがむくみますか？」
「次のようなときにひどく咳き込んだりしますか。空気が煙いとき，ほこりっぽいとき，あるいは寒い屋外に出るなどして，温度が変わるときなど。咳がひどくなる姿勢はありますか？」
「痰に血が混ざることはありますか？たくさん血液が混ざっていましたか，それとも血が線状に混ざっている程度ですか？」

Unit 4 COMMUNICATING

Some nursing/medical or Standard English words and corresponding colloquial words and expressions associated with communicating are given in Box. 2.

Note: Colloquial expressions used in the case histories and example conversations are explained in brackets [...].

BOX. 2
Words associated with communicating

Nursing/medical or Standard English words	Colloquial (everyday) or slang (very informal) words and expressions used by patients
Diplopia	Double vision; seeing double
Dysarthria[14]	Can't get the words out
Dysphasia (aphasia)	I know what to say but nothing comes out; I can't find the right word; the sentence comes out all wrong; I can say the word but I don't know what it means
Hearing impairment, deafness	Hard of hearing; deaf as a post
Tinnitus	Ringing, buzzing or roaring sound in the ears
Visual impairment, blindness	Can't see the hand in front of me; blind as a bat
Vertigo	Dizzy; dizziness; giddy

---

14. dysarthria「構音障害」意図した発音が正しくできない障害で,脳卒中の後遺症として残ることがある。

Unit 4　　　　　　　　　　　　　　　　　　　意思の疎通

意思の疎通に関連する看護・医学用語あるいは標準英語，対応する口語的な用語と表現を Box. 2 にまとめた。

注記：病歴と会話例文中における口語的な表現には，[　]内に説明を加えた。

BOX. 2

意思の疎通に関連する用語

看護/医学用語，または標準英語の用語	患者が使う口語的（日常的）または，俗語（非常にくだけた）用語と表現
複視	二重視，二重に見える
構音障害；運動障害性構音障害	言葉を発することができない
失語症	言いたいことはわかっているが言葉が1つも出ない；ちょうどよい言葉をみつけられない；文がまったくめちゃくちゃになって出る；言葉を発することはできるが意味は理解していない
難聴，聾	聞き取り困難；耳がまったく聞こえない
耳鳴り	音が鳴り響く感じ；耳の中でブンブンいう音やうなるような音がすること
視覚障害，盲（もう），失明	自分の前にある手が見えない；全然見えない
めまい	めまいがする；めまい；めまい

Case history 2 Speech problems due to a stroke: Mrs Egbewole

Mrs Egbewole had a stroke (cerebrovascular accident) about 18 months ago, and her family, with the help of twice-daily visits from the home carer, usually look after her at home. She has come into the care home while her family has a short holiday. The stroke has left Mrs Egbewole with left-sided paralysis and poor balance. She does not have dysphasia, but because the left side of her face is also paralysed she sometimes has slurred speech and dribbles saliva. She also has problems with nonverbal communication because her facial expression is affected.

3

Nurse: Mrs Egbewole, do you have any problems with your speech?

Mrs E.: It is slurred sometimes, but that's because my mouth doesn't work properly.

Nurse: How does that make you feel?

Mrs E.: I feel really embarrassed, especially if I'm talking to someone new.

Nurse: How can we help?

Mrs E.: I'll be all right as long as [provided] people give me enough time to get the words out. It gets me flustered [agitated/confused] if people are impatient.

Nurse: I'll make sure that is recorded in your care plan and that all members of staff know to give you plenty of time to tell us things. Did you see the speech and language therapist after the stroke?

Mrs E.: Yes, but I couldn't handle it [cope] so soon after losing my husband [my husband died].

Nurse: How would you feel about trying again with speech and language therapy?

Mrs E.: If you think it might help I'm willing to give it another go [try again].

★ 40

症例 2　　脳卒中による言語障害：エグベウォゥル夫人

エグベウォゥル夫人は18か月前に脳卒中（脳血管障害）を起こし，訪問介護士が1日2回やって来て手助けするほかは，通常家族が家で世話をしている。夫人は家族がちょっとした旅行に行く間，介護施設に来ている。脳卒中後，エグベウォゥル夫人は左半身麻痺となり，体のバランスが取りにくくなった。失語症にはなっていないものの，顔の左半分も麻痺しているため，言葉が不明瞭になったり，よだれが垂れたりすることがある。顔の表情に影響が出たため非言語的コミュニケーションにも問題がある。

看護師：　エグベウォゥルさん，話をするのに問題がありますか？

E夫人：　ときどきはっきり話せないことがあります。でもそれは，口がちゃんと動かないからです。

看護師：　そのことについてどう感じますか？

E夫人：　本当に気恥ずかしく感じます。特に，初めて会う人と話しているときには。

看護師：　どんなことが助けになりますか？

E夫人：　言葉をちゃんと話せるまで時間をいただければ［いただける限りは］大丈夫です。周りの人がもどかしそうにしていると，落ち着きません［動揺します，困惑します］。

看護師：　このことは必ず看護計画に書き，あなたが話すとき十分に時間をかけられるよう，スタッフみんなが知るようにします。脳卒中の後に言語療法士に診てもらましたか？

E夫人：　はい。でも主人を失った［主人が亡くなった］ばかりで手に負えませんでした［ついていけませんでした］。

看護師：　もう一度言語療法を受けてみてはいかがですか？

E夫人：　それが役立つとお考えでしたらもう1度やってみよう［試みよう］と思います。

Nurse: Fine — I'll organise a referral. Is there anything else that's troubling you?

Mrs E.: Well yes there is, and it's all down to [caused by] the muscles in my face not working properly. I can't help dribbling [saliva flows from the mouth].

Nurse: You obviously know about keeping the skin round your mouth clean and dry because there is no sign of soreness.

Mrs E.: Yes, the nurses on the stroke unit really stressed good skin care. But another thing that worries me is the look of my face – it's really lopsided [asymmetrical] and when I try to smile I must look dreadful.

Nurse: Maybe the speech and language therapist can suggest something to help, but you could mention it to Dr Newell. She will be in this afternoon.

Mrs E.: That's a good idea - I will add it to my list of questions I have for her.

Nurse: How is your sight? I see you have spectacles/glasses on at the moment.

Mrs E.: Yes, I'm blind as a bat without them [usually meaning poor vision rather than completely blind] and have needed help for years. I used to have contact lenses, but after my stroke I found it too difficult to take them out, so I got some specs [short for 'spectacles'].

Nurse: Do you have a second pair for reading or does the one pair do for everything?

Mrs E.: They are bifocals and I am supposed to look through a different bit for reading. But if the print is very small, such as on food labels, I use a magnifying glass instead.

Nurse: Did you bring the magnifying glass in with you?

Mrs E.: Oh yes, my carer packed everything but the kitchen sink [implies that the carer was very thorough when he packed Mrs Egbewole's suitcase].

看護師:	それがいいです ─ 紹介の準備をします。ほかにお困りのことはありますか？
E夫人:	そうですね，ええ，あります。顔の筋肉がうまく動かないせい［ことが原因］ですが，どうしてもよだれが垂れてしまいます［唾液が口から流れてしまいます］。
看護師:	ただれがありませんから，口の周りの皮膚を清潔にして乾かしておくことは間違いなくご存じのようですね。
E夫人:	はい。脳卒中で入院した病棟の看護師さんが正しい皮膚の手入れの大切さを強調していました。もう1つの心配事は，顔の外見です ─ すごくゆがんでいる［左右非対称な］ので，笑おうとすると本当にひどいでしょう。
看護師:	言語療法士が役に立つことを教えてくれるかもしれませんが，ニュウェル先生にお話しするのもいいかもしれません。先生は今日の午後来ます。
E夫人:	それがいいですね。先生への質問リストにこのことを加えます。
看護師:	視力の方はどうですか？今は眼鏡をかけていますね。
E夫人:	はい。眼鏡無しではまるで見えません［通常，まったく見えないのではなく視力が弱いことを意味する］し，ずいぶん前から補助が必要です。以前はコンタクトレンズを使っていましたが，卒中の後はあまりにもレンズを取り出しづらくなって，眼鏡［specs は spectacles「眼鏡」の略］を買いました。
看護師:	読書用に別の眼鏡をお持ちですか？それとも1つの眼鏡ですべてすませられますか？
E夫人:	これは遠近両用の眼鏡で，読むときは違うところを通して見るようになっています。でも，食品表示のラベルにあるような，とても小さい字には，代わりに拡大鏡を使います。
看護師:	拡大鏡も一緒にお持ちになりましたか？
E夫人:	はい。介護士さんが，台所の流し以外はみんな荷物に入れてくれました［介護士がエグベウォル夫人のスーツケースに荷物を詰める際，周到であったことを意味している］。

	Nurse:	Who normally cleans your spectacles?
55	Mrs E.:	My lovely [meaning admirable in this case] carers do that, I can't with only one good hand.
	Nurse:	Would you like me to give them a clean now?
	Mrs E.:	Thanks — they're not very clean and it makes things look blurred.
60	Nurse:	Do you have any other problems with your eyes? Sometimes a stroke can affect vision, such as seeing things double.
	Mrs E.:	Oh no, I was lucky [that the stroke did not affect her sight]. When I was younger I suffered terribly [very badly affected] with migraine and then I used to see flashing lights with a
65		zigzag pattern before the headache came on [started]. If I'm out in a cold wind my eyes start running [watering; tears flow down the cheeks], but that's normal.
	Nurse:	Definitely normal — it certainly happens to me.

Case history 3   Poor hearing and tinnitus: Mr Sandford

Mr Sandford is 42 years old and has poor hearing, tinnitus and problems with the build-up of earwax, which also affects his hearing. He has Down syndrome and lives independently at the local group housing complex where he has a bedsit. He works full-time in a supermarket.
His parents are dead, but his two older sisters, who live close by, see him several times a week and he has many friends from work and in the house.

	Nurse:	Hello Mr Sandford, I'm Nurse MacGregor. I understand that you have come to see us about your hearing.
	Mr S.:	Hello, everyone calls me Nick. My hearing is no good, I can't hear them on the telly[15] [television] or the boss [manager] at

---

15.telly「テレビ」英国の口語, television の略。

看護師：　　普段はだれが眼鏡をきれいにしていますか？

E夫人：　　私の愛すべき［ここではlovelyは「愛すべき」を意味する］介護士さんたちです。ちゃんと使える手片方だけではできませんから。

看護師：　　今私が眼鏡をきれいにしましょうか？

E夫人：　　ありがとうございます。あまりきれいではないので，ものがぼやけて見えます。

看護師：　　ほかに何か目の問題はありますか。脳卒中は目に影響することがあります。例えば，ものが二重に見えるといったような。

E夫人：　　いいえ。私は運が良かったです［脳卒中は視覚に影響しなかった］。若かったころは片頭痛にひどく悩まされて，頭痛が来る［始まる］前は，光がジグザグ模様にちらちら見えていました。〔今は〕冷たい風の吹く日に外に出ると涙が出ます［涙が流れる，涙が頬をつたい落ちる］。でもこれは普通のことですよね。

看護師：　　まったく普通のことです。私もそうなりますよ。

症例3　　聴力障害と耳鳴り：サンドフォード氏

　サンドフォード氏は42歳で，聴力が低く，耳鳴りがある。また，耳あかがたまる問題があり，それも聴力に影響を及ぼしている。彼はダウン症候群で，地域のグループハウスの一部屋で独立して暮らしている。スーパーで常勤で働いている。彼の両親は亡くなったが，近くに住む2人の姉が週に数回会いに来る。職場にもグループハウスにも，たくさん友人がいる。

看護師：　　こんにちはサンドフォードさん，私は看護師のマグレガーです。聴力の件でいらしたんですよね。

S氏：　　　こんにちは。みんなは私のことをニックと呼びます。聴力がだめで，テレビ［テレビ］の音やお店の上司［マネジャー］の声が聞こえません。

5		the shop.
	Nurse:	Can you hear me all right?
	Mr S.:	Yes.
	Nurse:	What would you like me to call you?
	Mr S.:	You can call me Nick if you like.
10	Nurse:	OK. Has your hearing always been bad Nick?
	Mr S.:	Not as bad – it's really bad now and I can't hear the telly.
	Nurse:	What do you like on the telly?
	Mr S.:	I watch Eastenders and Coronation Street [both popular, long-running series in the UK], they're the best and I like the
15		football as well.
	Nurse:	What helps you to hear?
	Mr S.:	Like now when I can see you and nobody else is talking. When I'm calm.
	Nurse:	Anything else?
20	Mr S.:	The ear wash [ear irrigation, previously known as 'syringing'] but it feels funny [strange].
	Nurse:	We can have a look inside your ears with the special light [otoscope] to check for wax, you might need another ear wash to help you hear.
25	Mr S.:	OK.
	Nurse:	Have you got a hearing aid?
	Mr S.:	Don't like it.
	Nurse:	What don't you like?
	Mr S.:	It's broken.
30	Nurse:	Have you got it with you? Perhaps the technician can mend it.
	Mr S.:	Here it is, but it's no good.
	Nurse:	I'll take it to the technician in a bit [in a short while]. Does anything else happen as well as not being able to hear?
35	Mr S.:	Roaring [loud noise] and buzzing [like the sound made by insects] in my ears.
	Nurse:	Anything else?

★ 46

看護師：	私の声は聞こえますか？
S氏：	はい。
看護師：	あなたをどのようにお呼びしましょう？
S氏：	ニックで結構です。
看護師：	わかりました。これまでもずっと耳の聞こえが悪かったのですか，ニック？
S氏：	それほどでも ― 今は本当に悪くてテレビが聞こえません。
看護師：	どんなテレビ番組が好きですか？
S氏：	イーストエンダーズとコロネイション・ストリート［両方とも英国で人気の長寿シリーズ］が1番です。サッカーも好きです。
看護師：	どうすると聞きききやすくなりますか？
S氏：	今のような感じです。話し相手が見えていて，ほかにだれも話していないとき，自分が落ち着いているときです。
看護師：	ほかには？
S氏：	耳を洗うこと［耳洗浄，以前は「シリンジング（耳洗浄）」として知られていた］ですが，奇妙な［変な］感じがします。
看護師：	特別なライト［耳鏡］を使って耳の中の耳あかを調べましょう。聞こえるようにするために，また耳洗浄が必要かもしれません。
S氏：	はい。
看護師：	補聴器はお持ちですか？
S氏：	好きじゃありません。
看護師：	どんなところが気に入らないのですか？
S氏：	壊れています。
看護師：	今持っていますか？たぶん技師が直せますよ。
S氏：	これです，でも役に立ちませんよ。
看護師：	それをちょっとしたら［間もなく］技師のところに持って行きます。聞こえないほかに，何かありますか？
S氏：	耳の中でうなるような音［大きな雑音］やブーンという音［虫の羽音のような音］がします。
看護師：	ほかには？

	Mr S.:	My ears feel stuffed up [fullness] and I get giddy [experience vertigo] and stagger.
40	Nurse:	Do you fall over?
	Mr S.:	I know it's coming, so I sit down.

S氏：　　　両耳が詰まっている［いっぱいになっている］感じがして，めまいがし［めまいを経験し］，足がよろよろします。
看護師：　倒れますか？
S氏：　　　倒れそうになるのがわかるので，座ります。

Unit 5   SAFETY AND PREVENTING ACCIDENTS

Some nursing/medical or Standard English words and corresponding colloquial words and expressions associated with safety and preventing accidents are given in Box. 3.

Note: Colloquial expressions used in the case histories and example conversations are explained in brackets [...].

BOX. 3
Words associated with safety and preventing accidents

Nursing/medical or Standard English words	Colloquial (everyday) or slang (very informal) words and expressions used by patients
Fall	Took a tumble; lost my footing; tripped up
Fracture	Broken or cracked (as in bone)
Seizure	Fit; funny turn; convulsion; an attack
Sprain	Twisted (as in ankle)
Syncope	Fainting attack; black out; collapse; pass out
Unconscious	Knocked out (KO'd); out cold; dead to the world; out of it

Case history 4   A scald: Mrs Kaur

Mrs Kaur has scalded her arm while making a cup of tea. Her neighbour brought her to the Emergency Department after they had bathed the damaged area with lots of cool water and kept it cool on the way to hospital with a wet towel. She is upset about being so clumsy
5   and feels that she has been a nuisance to her neighbour and to the hospital staff who already have enough to do. Luckily the skin damage is superficial and should be completely healed in a few days.

Unit 5　　　　　　　　　　　　　　　　安全と事故防止

安全と事故防止に関連する看護・医学用語あるいは標準英語，対応する口語的な用語と表現を Box. 3 にまとめた。

注記：病歴と会話例文中における口語的な表現には，〔　〕内に説明を加えた。

BOX. 3

安全と事故防止に関連する用語

看護／医学用語， または標準英語の用語	患者が使う口語的（日常的） または，俗語（非常にくだけた）単語と表現
転倒	ころんだ；足をすべらせた；つまずいた
骨折	（骨を）折った；（骨に）ひびが入った
けいれん，発作	発作，ひきつけ；けいれん；発作
捻挫	ひねった（足首など）
失神	気絶；〔一時的な〕意識不明；卒倒
意識不明の	気絶した（KO'd とも表記）；無意識の〔主に頭に打撃を受けて〕；意識もなくて；〔疲労・薬・アルコールで〕もうろうとして

症例 4　　（熱湯による）やけど：カウア夫人

カウア夫人は，お茶を用意しているときに腕をやけどした。近所の人たちが大量の冷たい水でやけどの場所を洗った後，濡れタオルで冷やしながら，病院の救急科に連れてきた。彼女はこのような不始末をしたことに動揺しており，近所の人や多忙な病院のスタッフを煩わせてしまっていると感じている。幸い皮膚の損傷は浅いものであり，数日ですっかり良くなるはずである。

Nurse:	Hello again Mrs Kaur. Have the painkillers worked [taken away the pain]?
Mrs K.:	Hello Nurse. Yes, the pain is much less. My arm just feels sore [tender].
Nurse:	The plan is to keep the scald dry and warm and let it heal. I've come to put a dressing on your arm.
Mrs K.:	I don't want anything that will stick.
Nurse:	The dressings we use don't stick anymore, they are made to be non-adherent.
Mrs K.:	I remember the pain years ago when dressings did stick.
Nurse:	The dressing only needs to be on for a few days and the scald will heal. It was a good thing that you knew the first aid for scalds, cooling the skin down certainly stopped it getting any worse.
Mrs K.:	I saw a thing on the telly [television] about what to do with burns. But what about some burn ointment? It must need something.
Nurse:	If you leave the dressing on for 2 or 3 days the scald will heal without any other treatment. You can take mild painkillers such as paracetamol[16] if your arm is sore.
Mrs K.:	I don't like the idea of taking it [the dressing] off myself.
Nurse:	Well today is Saturday, so it should all be healed by Monday. You can get an appointment with the practice nurse for Tuesday and she can take off the dressing and check your arm.
Mrs K.:	Sounds sensible — I will do that. I really feel such a fool — how could I pour boiling water over myself. I am doing all the silly things my granny [grandmother] did when she was 80.
Nurse:	How do you think it happened?

---

16. paracetamol「パラセタモール」非アスピリン系解熱・鎮痛薬。日本や米国ではacetaminophen「アセトアミノフェン」と呼ばれる。

看護師： また来ましたよ，カウアさん。痛み止めは効いていますか［痛みを取り除きましたか］？

Kさん： 看護師さん，こんにちは。はい，痛みはだいぶ良くなりました。腕はひりひりする［触れると痛む］だけです。

看護師： 計画では，やけどを乾かして暖かくしておいて，自然に治るようにします。腕に包帯を巻きに来ましたよ。

Kさん： くっついてしまうものはいやなのですが。

看護師： ここで使っている包帯はくっつくことはないですよ。非粘着性にできています。

Kさん： 何年か前，包帯がくっついてすごく痛かったのを覚えています。

看護師： 包帯が必要なのは数日の間だけで，それでやけどは治りますよ。やけどの応急処置を知っていらしてよかったです。皮膚を冷やしておくと確実にそれ以上悪くならなくてすみますから。

Kさん： テレビ［テレビ］でやけどしたらどうしたらよいか見ました。だけど，やけど用の塗り薬はどうですか。何かつけなければならないでしょう。

看護師： 2，3日包帯を巻いておいたら，ほかには治療をしなくてもやけどは治りますよ。もし腕がひりひり痛むようなら，パラセタモールのような強くない鎮痛薬を飲むといいです。

Kさん： 自分でこれ［包帯］を外したくないのですが。

看護師： えーと，今日は土曜日ですから，月曜日にはすっかり良くなっているでしょう。火曜日に開業看護師の予約がとれますから，包帯を外して腕を見てもらいましょう。

Kさん： よさそうですね。そうします。本当に馬鹿だなと思います ― 熱湯を自分にかけてしまうなんて。おばあちゃん［祖母］が80歳のときにやっていた馬鹿げたことすべてをしているのです。

看護師： どういう風にしてやけどしたと思いますか？

	Mrs K.:	I can't seem to judge where the cup is. It's the same when I pour orange juice into a glass. And the kettle is so heavy.
	Nurse:	Have you had your eyes checked recently?
35	Mrs K.:	My routine test must be due very soon — I will phone on Monday.
	Nurse:	Could you talk to the practice nurse about the trouble [difficulty] you have when pouring fluids?
	Mrs K.:	Yes, do you think I should tell her about how things are blurred and sometimes lines look very odd and wavy?
40	Nurse:	That sounds like a good idea. But what can you do to make the kettle easier to use?
	Mrs K.:	I forget it's only me having a drink and usually fill it too full.
	Nurse:	Yes, I just fill mine without thinking. I have seen smaller kettles. Perhaps you would find that easier.
45	Mrs K.:	My daughter can get me one when she goes to the big shops.

Case history 5   Instructions on the use of drugs: Mr Anderson

Mr Anderson is going home with several different drugs. He has been in hospital to have intravenous antibiotics for cellulitis and needs to have a course of oral antibiotics (phenoxymethylpenicillin, flucloxacillin and metronidazole). He also takes an antiepileptic drug (sodium valproate) to control generalised seizures and a diuretic (torasemide) for hypertension.

🔊 6

Nurse: The antibiotics for you to take home have come up from the pharmacy and I would like to go over [discuss] what

Kさん：	カップがどこにあるのかよくわかっていないんだと思います。オレンジ・ジュースをコップに注ぐときにもそういうことがあります。おまけに，やかんはとても重いですし。
看護師：	最近眼の検査を受けましたか？
Kさん：	もうすぐ定期健診のはずです。月曜日に電話してみます。
看護師：	開業看護師に，液体を注ぐときの問題［困難さ］について話していただけますか？
Kさん：	はい。どのように物がぼやけて見えるかとか，ときどき線が奇妙に見えたり，波打って見えたりすることも話した方がいいと思いますか？
看護師：	それはいい考えですね。どうしたらやかんが使いやすくなると思いますか？
Kさん：	飲むのは私1人だということを忘れて，たいてい〔やかんを〕いっぱいにしてしまうんです。
看護師：	ええ，私も何も考えないで入れています。小型のやかんを見たことがあります。それだともっと簡単かもしれませんよ。
Kさん：	娘が大型店に行ったときに買ってきてもらえます。

症例5　　　服薬指導：アンダーソン氏

アンダーソン氏は何種類かの薬を持って退院するところである。入院中，彼は蜂巣炎治療のために静脈からの抗生物質投与を受けていた。今後さらに，1クールの，経口による抗生物質（フェノキシメチルペニシリン，フルクロキサシリン，メトロニダゾール）投与が必要である。彼はまた，てんかんの全般発作を抑えるために抗てんかん薬（バルプロ酸ナトリウム）を，高血圧のために利尿薬（トラセミド）を服用している。

看護師：	薬剤部から家に持ち帰っていただく抗生物質が届きましたので，これからやっていただきたいことを説明します［話します］。ラベルに指

		you need to do. There are instructions on the labels, but it helps if we talk it through [discuss] as well.
5	Mr A.:	Yeah [yes], OK then. I want to get it right. It was a bit of a fright ending up in here just for a cat bite gone septic [infected].
	Nurse:	What seems like such a minor thing can quickly get really bad. There are three separate antibiotics to take - here look [at the containers]. There are two penicillins: flucloxacillin[17] and phenoxymethylpenicillin. You need to take these every 6 hours and an hour before food or on an empty stomach. These are the best ones for your infection and you have already told us that you are not allergic to penicillin. The other antibiotic is metronidazole[18], which you need to take every 8 hours, but this time with or after food.
	Mr A.:	Yeah, no problems with penicillin and I'm used to taking tablets — with the Epilim [a proprietary name for sodium valproate[19]] twice a day and the Torem [proprietary name for torasemide[20]] first thing [earlymorning].
	Nurse:	Will there be any problem with having to take two before food and one with or after food?
	Mr A.:	No, I already need to remember to take the Epilim after food.
25	Nurse:	What about writing out a chart? That would help, especially if you cross off doses as you take them.
	Mr A.:	I don't write so well, but one of our kids [children] can do it.
	Nurse:	It is important to take the antibiotics at regular times and to finish the 7-day course even if your hand seems better.
30	Mr A.:	Why can't I stop once it looks better?

---

17. flucloxacillin「フルクロキサシリン」外傷または肺炎などの連鎖球菌性感染症の治療に使われるペニシリン薬。
18. metronidazole「メトロニダゾール」抗トリコモナス薬, 服用中にアルコールを摂取するとひどい悪酔いを引き起こす抗菌薬。
19. valproate「バルプロ酸ナトリウム」抗けいれん剤。
20. torasemide「トラセミド」ループ利尿薬。

	示が書いてありますが，ここで洗いざらい話して［話し合って］おくと役に立つでしょう。
A氏：	ええ［はい］，わかりました。きちんと理解しておきたいです。ただ猫にかまれたところが，化膿［感染］してここ〔病院〕に行きつくなんてちょっと怖いことでしたよ。
看護師：	とてもささいに見えることが，あっという間に非常に悪いことになってしまうことがありますね。3種類のそれぞれ異なる抗生物質が出ています ―［入れ物を］見てください。ペニシリンが2種類 ― フルクロキサシリンとフェノキシメチルペニシリン。この2種類を6時間ごとに，食事の1時間前か空腹時に飲む必要があります。あなたの感染症にはこの2つが一番よく効きます。ペニシリンにアレルギーがないということはすでにお聞きしていますね。もう1つの抗生物質はメトロニダゾールで，こちらは8時間ごと，食事中または食後に飲む必要があります。
A氏：	ええ，ペニシリンは問題ないですし，錠剤を飲むのにも慣れています。エピリム［バルプロ酸ナトリウムの登録商標名］を1日2回，トレム［torasemide「トラセミド」の登録商標名］を朝一番［早朝］に飲んでます。
看護師：	食前に2種類，そして食後に1種類飲まなければならないのは問題になりますか？
A氏：	いいえ，以前から食後にエピリムを飲むのを忘れないようにしなければなりませんから。
看護師：	表に書き込んだらどうでしょう。役に立つと思いますよ。特に，飲むたびに線を引いていくといいと思います。
A氏：	私はそういうものを書くのがうまくないですが，うちの子［子供］の1人ができると思います。
看護師：	大事なのは，決まった時間に抗生物質を飲むこと，そして手の具合が良くなってきているようでも7日間飲み続けることです。
A氏：	良くなったようでも止めてはいけないのはどうしてですか？

	Nurse:	Finishing the course means that the treatment will kill off all the bugs [bacteria in this case] — the infection is cured, and it is very important the bugs don't become immune [develop resistance] to the antibiotics.
35	Mr A.:	What like that MRSA[21] has? OK. I'll carry on [continue] to the end.
	Nurse:	Yes, just like MRSA, but you haven't got that. There are a few other things I need to tell you about the metronidazole. It is important to swallow the tablets whole with plenty of water. And you shouldn't drink alcohol while you are taking them and for 2 days after you stop — it can cause a nasty reaction with nausea and sickness [vomiting]. You might have a furred tongue and your urine can be dark.
45	Mr A.:	That's a blow [disappointment]. I could really do with[22] a couple of pints [meaning he would enjoy some beer]. Thanks for the warning about my pee [urine]. That would have really put the wind up[23] me [alarm me].
	Nurse:	Have you got plenty of Epilim and Torem at home?
50	Mr A.:	Yeah — I never run out of tablets [have none left]. I dread having another fit [seizure] now that they have settled down.
	Nurse:	Have you any questions or bits you don't quite understand?
	Mr A.:	It's a lot to take in [information to absorb, understand]. Can you go through it all again please?
55	Nurse:	You're right it is a lot of information. Let's start with the three antibiotics and when to take them ...

---

21. MRSA「メシチリン耐性黄色ブドウ球菌」methicillin-resistant *Staphylococcus aureus* の略。
22. could do with ... = would be glad to have ...「〜があればありがたい, 欲しい, 必要である」
23. put the wind up ... 「〜を怖がらせる, 不安がらせる」

看護師：	決められたように抗生物質を飲み終えるということは，その治療ですべてのばい菌［この場合は細菌］を駆除するということです ─ それで感染症は治ります。とても大事なのは，ばい菌が抗生物質の効かない菌になってしまう［耐性が生じる］ことがないようにすることです。
A 氏：	MRSA にかかった時みたいにですか？わかりました。最後まで続け［継続し］ます。
看護師：	そうです，MRSA のようにです。これにはかかりませんでしたけどね。メトロニダゾールについて，ほかにもいくつかお話しておくべきことがあります。大切なのは，たくさんの水で錠剤を丸ごと飲むことです。それから，この薬を飲んでいる間と飲み終えてからの 2 日間はお酒を飲んではいけません。胸のむかつきや吐き気［嘔吐］といった不快な反応を起こすことがあります。舌ごけが出ることもありますし，尿の色が濃くなることもありますね。
A 氏：	それはショック［残念］です。2, 3 杯飲めたらありがたいですけどね［ビールを楽しむことを意味する］。おしっこ［尿］について警告してくださってありがとう。尿に異常が出るなんて不安になります［警戒します］からね。
看護師：	家にエピレムとトレムはたくさんありますか？
A 氏：	ええ ─ 薬を切らしたことはありません［錠剤がなくなったことはありません］。発作が落ち着いているので，また発作［発作］が出るのは怖いです。
看護師：	質問や，よくわからないところはありますか？
A 氏：	のみ込まなければならないこと［吸収するべき情報，理解しなければならないこと］がたくさんですね。もう一度繰り返していただけますか？
看護師：	おっしゃる通り，情報がたくさんです。3 種類の抗生物質をいつ飲むかから始めましょう…。

Unit 6   MOBILITY

Some nursing/medical or Standard English words and corresponding colloquial words and expressions associated with mobility are given in Box. 4.

Note: Colloquial expressions used in the case histories and example conversations are explained in brackets [...].

BOX. 4

Words associated with mobility

Nursing/medical or Standard English words	Colloquial (everyday) or slang (very informal) words and expressions used by patients
Akinesia	Freezing or frozen; rooted to the Spot; can't go forward
Ataxia[24]	Staggering; jerky; shaky; all over the place
Bradykinesia[25]	Can't get started; slowed me almost to a halt; slowed me down nearly to a complete stop
Dorsal part of a phalangeal joint, especially the metacarpophalangeal joints[26] (with fingers flexed)	Knuckle
Sudden tonic muscle contraction	Cramp
Festination	Shuffling; can't stop once I get going
Swollen	Puffed up
Swollen and deformed (as an arthritic finger joint) Tremor[27]	Knobbly The shakes

---

24.ataxia「運動失調, 失調」随意運動中の筋活動を協調させられないこと。小脳または脊髄後索の疾患によるものが多い。肢, 頭, または体幹を侵す。
25.bradykinesia「運動緩徐」自発性と運動の減少。パーキンソン病などの錐体外路性疾患の症状のひとつ。
26.metacarpophalangeal joint「中手指節関節」中手骨頭は掌側から見ると不完全に二分されているためこの関節は2つの顆状関節のように見える。
27.tremor「振戦」①反復性でしばしば規則性の震える運動。対立筋群の交代性または同期性の不規則収縮による。通常不随意性。②物を注視している間に起こる眼球のかすかな動き。

Unit 6　運動能力

運動能力に関連する看護・医学用語あるいは標準英語，対応する口語的な用語と表現を Box. 4 にまとめた。

注記：病歴と会話例文中における口語的な表現には，[　]内に説明を加えた。

BOX. 4

運動能力に関連した語

看護・医療用語 または標準的な用語	患者が使う口語的（日常的） または，俗語の（非常にくだけた）用語と表現
失動〔運動不能〕	すくんで，身動きできなくて，釘付けになって，前に進むことができない
運動失調〔失調〕	千鳥足の，ぎくしゃくした，よろめいた，抑えがきかなくなる
運動緩慢	始めることができない，ほとんど停止しそうなほど遅くなる，ほとんど完全に止るほど動きが鈍くなる
指節間関節の背側部，特に中手指節関節（指を屈曲させたとき）	指関節
突然の強直性筋収縮	けいれん
加速歩行（加速歩調）	すり足〔足を引きずること〕，一度進み始めると止められない
腫脹した	腫れた
腫れて変形した（関節炎の指関節のように）	瘤状の
振戦	震え

Case history 6   Rheumatoid arthritis: Ms Wayne

Joint stiffness and pain are causing Ms Wayne severe difficulties with mobility. She has had rheumatoid arthritis for many years and now has some joint destruction and deformity with associated muscle wasting. At the moment she feels generally unwell — very lethargic, her temperature is slightly elevated and she has anorexia. In the past she has had surgery to her hands, which are very badly affected.

7

Ms W.: Hello Nurse. Have you sorted out[28] [organised] my physiotherapy appointment yet?

Nurse: Yes, the physiotherapist is coming to treat you here. What do they usually do?

Ms W.: In the past I had heat treatment, but now they concentrate on gentle exercise and making sure that my hand splints are still helping and not making my skin sore.

Nurse: Tell me how your mobility is affected by the arthritis.

Ms W.: I have trouble [difficulties] getting in and out of bed, or the bath, and I need help to get out of a low chair.

Nurse: What about walking?

Ms W.: Getting about [moving about, going out] is hard. I get around the house with the walking aid[29] and tend to use a wheelchair when I go out. The car has been modified so at least I'm independent. I can go shopping and out with my pals [friends].

Nurse: Yes, that is important.

Ms W.: I'm not going to be an invalid [someone who is always ill], always needing help and griping [complaining] about the unfairness of it all.

Nurse: How do you stay so positive?

28. sort out「考えをまとめる」
29. walking aid「歩行器, 歩行補助道具」

症例6　　　関節リウマチ：ウェインさん

関節硬直と痛みのため，ウェインさんは運動能力に重大な障害をきたしている。彼女は何年もの間，関節リウマチを患っており，現在は関節破壊と変形が筋消耗を随伴して起こっている。現在のところ，彼女は概して気分がすぐれない — 無気力で微熱があり，食欲不振である。過去に両手に手術をしており，その具合がひどく悪くなっている。

Wさん：　こんにちは，看護師さん。理学療法士との予約をうまく取って［準備して］くださいましたか？

看護師：　はい，理学療法士は治療にここに来ることになっています。普段はどんな治療をしていますか？

Wさん：　以前は温熱治療でしたが，今は軽い運動に専念しています。手の添え木〔副子〕がまだうまく機能していて，それが皮膚をただれさせないように確認しながら〔軽い運動を〕しています。

看護師：　関節炎が動きにどう影響しているか話してください。

Wさん：　ベッドに寝るときと起きるとき，入浴のときが大変［難しい］です。それから，低い椅子から立ち上がるときには助けが必要です。

看護師：　歩行はどうですか？

Wさん：　歩き回る［動き回る，出歩く］のはつらいです。家の中では歩行補助具を使って動きますし，外出にはだいたい車椅子を使います。車を改造してもらったので，少なくとも自立はできています。買物に行ったり，友だち［友人］と出かけたりもできます。

看護師：　ええ，そういうことは重要ですね。

Wさん：　私はいつも助けを求めていて，こういった不公平にぶつぶつ言ってばかりいる［不平を言う］病人［いつも具合の悪い人］にはならないと決めているのです。

看護師：　どうやってそんなに前向きにしているのですか？

	Ms W.:	After my joints, especially my hands, got really bad [deteriorated] and I had to give up work [left employment] I thought 'I'm only 40 and can't just do nothing'. So I looked at ways I could be busy and useful.
	Nurse:	What do you do?
	Ms W.:	I go into the local primary school three mornings a week and listen to the children read. It's a great [good] feeling when you hear them improve and become more confident. Just lately I started helping on a telephone helpline for people with disabilities — there are special hands-free phones so I don't need to use my hands much.
	Nurse:	We [meaning Ms Wayne and the nurse] can sort out your care plan now and make sure that we include the help you need. You must tell me your usual routine for the hand splints, as you're the expert. Can you arrange for your own wheelchair to be brought in?
	Ms W.:	My brother can fetch[30] it at lunchtime if I give him a ring [contact by telephone].
	Nurse:	What about other activities? Do you have difficulty using your hands?
	Ms W.:	Yes, the pain and stiffness in my hands and wrists really hold me back [curb or inhibit]. My hands look so awful with the finger joints all puffed up [swollen] and it's so frustrating and it really riles [annoys, makes me angry] me when I can't do something simple like doing up [fastening] buttons. It's always worse in the morning when you need to wash and dress, which is a real pain [nuisance] when I'm due at the school.
	Nurse:	Are there any other movements that you find difficult?
	Ms W.:	Anything where I have to grip and move my wrist like holding the kettle and pouring.

30.fetch「取ってくる」

Wさん:	関節，特に手がとても悪くなった［悪化した］後，私は仕事を辞めなければ［職を辞さなければ］ならなくて，「まだ40歳なのにまったく何もできない」と思いました。それで私は忙しく有意義に過ごせる方法を考えたのです。
看護師:	どんなことをしていますか？
Wさん:	1週間に3日，午前中に地元の小学校に行って，子供たちが本を（声に出して）読むのを聞きます。子供たちが上手になって自信をつけるのを聞くとすばらしい［よい］気持ちになります。つい最近，障害を持つ人の電話相談の手伝いを始めました。そこにはハンズフリーの電話器があるので，そんなに手を使わなくてすみます。
看護師:	私たち［ウェインさんと看護師のこと］はこれから看護計画を調整して，必要な補助がきちんと含まれているか確認しましょう。よくご存じのあなたが普段手の添え木に何をしているのか説明してくださいね。ご自身の車椅子を持ってくるよう手配できますか？
Wさん:	はい，電話［電話を使って連絡］すれば，お昼の時間に兄弟に車椅子を取ってきてもらえます。
看護師:	ほかの動作についてはいかがでしょう。手を使うのは大変ですか？
Wさん:	はい，手と手首にある痛みとこわばりのせいで，いろいろとおっくうになります［抑制します，または，妨げになります］。指関節がすべて腫れて［むくんで］いて手がとても見苦しいですし。ボタンを掛ける［留める］ような簡単なことができないとき，とてもいらいらしてもどかしいです［むかむかします，腹が立ちます］。朝，顔を洗ったり，身支度を整えなければならないときにいつも悪くなるのです，学校に行くことになっているときには本当にいやに［不愉快に］なります。
看護師:	ほかに難しいと感じる動作はありますか？
Wさん:	やかんを握って注ぐというような，何かを握って手首を動かすことなら何でも。

	Nurse:	Again we can plan what help you will need from us while you're here. Do you see the OT [occupational therapist] for help with this?
	Ms W.:	Yes, she has been so helpful — lots of gadgets to help me do things, like dressing and cooking, for myself, and so many good ideas about how to do things without getting tired or making the pain worse.
	Nurse:	Perhaps your brother can bring in the gadgets you need in here when he comes with the wheelchair. What do you think?
	Ms W.:	OK. I hadn't thought of that.
	Nurse:	The rheumatology nurse specialist[31] will be up later to review your drugs with Dr Wong [the rheumatologist], and co-ordinate all the other practitioners — I expect you know them both quite well by now.
	Ms W.:	Yes, I certainly do. Having Sam [Ms Wayne has known the nurse specialist for several years and they use first names] is a real support — he's always there on the phone and it's so nice to see the same person at the nurse-led clinics[32]. I'm a bit disappointed about the new drugs we tried — the benefits have definitely worn off [become less effective].
	Nurse:	Do you need anything for pain?
	Ms W.:	No, not at the moment thanks. I took all my morning drugs at home and I'd rather wait to see what happens after the drug review.

---

31. rheumatology nurse specialist「リウマチ専門看護師」英国では，国の定めた条件（経験，学業など）をみたすことで，希望する専門分野の職務領域を広げることができる。
32. nurse-led clinic「看護師主導診療所」各診療所により異なるが，多くは上級看護師により運営され，診断，病歴の聴取，病状の観察，薬剤の処方などを行う。

看護師: 繰り返しになりますが，あなたがここにいる間に，どんな助けが必要になるか計画を立てましょう。〔改善の〕助けになるように OT［作業療法士］に診てもらっていますか？

Wさん: はい，彼女はとても協力的です。自分で服を着たり料理をしたりという，何かをするのに役に立つ気の利いた道具や，疲れや痛みをひどくしないでいろいろなことをできる方法について，とてもたくさんの良いアイデアをくれます。

看護師: 兄弟の方に，ここで必要な道具をいくつか，車椅子と一緒に持ってきてもらいましょう。いかがですか？

Wさん: お願いします。考えもしませんでした。

看護師: 後で，リウマチ専門看護師がウオン先生［リウマチ専門医］と一緒に処方薬の見直しに来ます。そして，ほかの専門家たちみんなの調整をします。彼ら2人のことはもうよくご存知でしょう。

Wさん: はい，もちろんです。サム［ウエインさんはその専門看護師をもう何年も知っており，ファーストネームで呼び合っている］はとても支えになってくれています。いつも電話に出てくれるし，看護師主導診療所で顔見知りに会えるのはとてもうれしいです。私たちが試した新しい薬にはちょっとがっかりしましたけど。明らかに効果が切れてきましたので［効果が減少したので］。

看護師: 痛み止めは必要ですか？

Wさん: いいえ，今は結構です。家で朝の薬をすべて飲んできたので，薬の見直しをした後，どうなるか待ちたいと思います。

Case history 7   Parkinson's disease: Mr Lajowski

Mr Lajowski has come into the day-surgery unit to have a lipoma removed from his back. His mobility is seriously affected by Parkinson's disease, which he has had for some years. He is not particularly anxious about the surgery, as this was explained to him at the pre-admission
5   assessment clinic[33], but he is worried about how he will cope with moving about[34] in the new environment.

Nurse: Hello Mr Lajowski. I understand that you have come in today to have a fatty lump [lipoma] removed from your back and the plan is to send you home later this afternoon.

Mr L.: Yes, that's right. The lump needs to come off [be removed]
5   — it gets in the way of the waistband of my trousers. I shall be glad to see the back of it [pleased when it has gone]. Did they tell you that I have Parkinson's disease?

Nurse: Yes, it's in your notes from the assessment clinic. How does it affect you?

10 Mr L.: The walking is the worst. Its difficult to start moving and I'm so slow [bradykinesia]. All I can do is shuffle [feet sliding, legs dragging, characteristic of Parkinson's disease] to start with and then my steps get shorter and I get faster and faster [festination[35]], can't stop, and like as not [likely] over
15   I go [fall over]. I've really lost my nerve [to lose confidence]. If you saw me you would think I was the worse for drink ['drink' in this case means alcoholic drink — the person is drunk, or intoxicated, or inebriated].

Nurse: Do you have any other movement problems?

20 Mr L.: I get that freezing [akinesia] where I'm rooted to the spot

---
33. pre-admission assessment clinic 「術前検査外来」手術内容などについての説明や、アレルギーなどの検査をあらかじめ受ける。
34. move about 「あちこち動きまわる」
35. festination 「歩行強迫, 加速歩行」無意識に歩行が速くなる。

症例6　　パーキンソン病：ラジャウスキ氏

ラジャウスキ氏は，脂肪腫を背中から取り除くために日帰り手術病棟に来た。ここ数年患っているパーキンソン病によって運動能力が深刻な影響を受けている。術前検査外来で説明を受けたので手術については特に心配はしていないが，よく知らない環境でどうしたらうまく動き回れるか心配している。

看護師：　こんにちは，ラジャウスキさん。今日は，背中の脂肪性の腫瘍［脂肪腫］の除去のために来て，午後には家に帰る予定ですね。

L氏：　　はい，その通りです。脂肪腫を取って［取り除いて］もらわないと。脂肪腫はズボンのウエストベルトの邪魔になるんです。取れたらせいせいしますよ［なくなったらうれしいです］。私がパーキンソン病なのはお聞きですか？

看護師：　はい，術前検査外来からのメモに書いてあります。〔パーキンソン病で〕どのような影響がありますか？

L氏：　　歩行が1番悪いです。動き始めるのが大変で，とても遅い［運動緩慢］です。最初はすり足でゆっくりと歩く［足を引きずって歩く，パーキンソン病に特徴的な症状］ことしかできず，それから歩幅が短くなってどんどん速く［加速歩行に］なり，止まることができなくてだいたいは［ほとんど］ひっくり返りそうになります［倒れそうになります］。本当に度胸［自信］を失くしています。もしあなたが見たら，私は酒に酔っている［worse for drink「酔っている」ここでは drink はアルコールを意味する ─ 人が酔っぱらっている，酔っている，酒を飲み過ぎた］と思うでしょう。

看護師：　ほかにも動作障害がありますか？

L氏：　　足が釘付けになり［動けなくなり］，硬直してしまいます［無運動になります］。だいたいは思いがけなく［突然に］起こります。でも，1つ以上のことを1度に［同時］にしようとするせいで起こる［のが原因］

[can't move]. It mostly comes on out of the blue [comes unexpectedly], but I worked it out [found out, realised] that trying to do more than one thing at once [simultaneously] will bring it on [cause it]. The shaking [tremor] in my hands is bad, and its hard to do some things because my arms are so stiff [caused by rigidity].

Nurse: What things are particularly difficult for you?

Mr L.: It sounds daft [absurd], but it's mainly things like turning over in bed, reaching out for a cup, getting up out of a chair and turning round once I'm up.

Nurse: Are there things that help?

Mr L.: I've learnt a few tricks [ways to overcome the problems], such as having a good firm mattress and a high-backed chair with arms. The others things are really simple, like other people waiting until I'm ready to move and giving me time to do things for myself. When I freeze, the physio' [physiotherapist] told me to try stepping over an imaginary line, or to count 'one-two' out loud with each step and that does help.

Nurse: What about other activities, such as those needing fine movements?

Mr L.: Doing up [fastening] shoelaces or buttons is impossible, so that material that sticks to itself is very handy [helpful, useful]. What's it called again?

Nurse: Oh, you mean Velcro. It's very useful, we use it a lot in the rehab. [rehabilitation] unit.

Mr L.: I get loads [a lot] of cramp [sudden tonic muscle Contraction] attacks at night, so I'm awake half the night [disturbed sleep]. Before the Parkinson's I could just pop out [get out] of bed and it would go.

Nurse: Not so easy now.

Mr L.: How right you are. I wish it would settle down [become

だと思いつきました [知りました, 気がつきました]。手の震え [振戦] がひどくて, それから, 腕がとても硬い [硬直している] ので, 何かをするのが大変です。

看護師: どういうことが特に難しいですか？

L氏: おかしなこと [ばかげている] でしょうが, 主に, ベッドで寝がえりをうつ, カップに手を伸ばす, 椅子から立ち上がる, 立ち上がってから方向を変える, といったようなことです。

看護師: 助けになることはありますか。

L氏: いくつかコツ [問題を解決をする方法] をつかみました。マットレスをちゃんとした硬いものにしたり, 椅子を背もたれが高くてひじ掛のついたものにしたりというような。ほかはとても単純なことです。動く準備ができるまでほかの人に待ってもらう, 自分でできるように時間をもらう, といったようなことです。硬直したときには, 線があると想像して, それをまたぐようにするか, 一歩ごとに「1, 2」と声を出して数えるように理学療法士 [physio' は physiotherapist「理学療法士」の略] に言われています。それは助けになります。

看護師: 微細運動を必要とするような, ほかの動作はいかがですか？

L氏: 靴ひもを結んだり, ボタンをかける [しめる] のはまったくだめです。なので自然にくっつく素材のものはとても扱いやすいですね [役に立ちます, 便利です]。何というのでしたっけ？

看護師: ああ, ベルクロのことですね。とても便利で, リハビリ [rehab. は rehabilitation「リハビリテーション」の略] の病棟でたくさん使われています。

L氏: 夜中にたくさん [何度も] けいれん [突然の筋肉の収縮の発作] が起こり, そのせいで夜中まで目が覚めています [睡眠障害]。パーキンソン病になる前は, ベッドから抜け出せば [起き上れば] けいれんがおさまっていました。

看護師: 今はそんなに簡単ではありませんね。

L氏: 本当にその通りですよ。治まって [おとなしくなって休止して] くれればいいのですが。

	quiescent].
Nurse:	I gather [understand] that your medication has just [recently] been changed.
Mr L.:	Yes, I said to the Doc [short for doctor] that the cramp had gone on [continued] too long and he said that I could try some different tablets.
Nurse:	Any luck with the new tablets [meaning are they effective]?
Mr L.:	Early days [too soon to be sure], but I think the cramps have eased off [become less frequent].

看護師：	つい最近［最近］投薬治療が変わったばかりのようですね［と聞いています］。
L氏：	はい，医者［Docはdoctor「医師」の略］にけいれんが続く［継続する］のが長すぎると伝えたところ，違う薬を試してみようと言ったのです。
看護師：	新しい薬はうまくいっていますか［効果がありますか］？
L氏：	まだ早すぎます［時期尚早です］が，けいれんは和らいだ［そんなに頻繁ではなくなった］と思います。

Unit 7　EATING AND DRINKING

Some nursing/medical or Standard English words and corresponding colloquial words and expressions associated with eating and drinking are given in Box. 5.

Note: Colloquial expressions used in the case histories and example conversations are explained in brackets […].

BOX. 5
Words associated with eating and drinking

Nursing/medical or Standard English words	Colloquial (everyday) or slang (very informal) words and expressions used by patients
Abdomen[36]	Belly; gut[37]; stomach; tummy
Abdominal pain	Belly ache; gut rot; stomach/tummy ache
Anorexia	No appetite
Dyspepsia[38]	Acid indigestion; heartburn
Good appetite	Always hungry; eat like a horse; ready for my grub
Halitosis	Bad breath; mouth odour
Nausea	Biliousness; feel sick; queasiness
Oesophagus[39]	Gullet
Poor appetite	Can't face food; don't eat enough to keep a bird alive; been off my food; not hungry; peck or pick at food
Stomatitis	Mouth ulcers; sore mouth
Vomit	Be sick; bring up; lose the lot; puke; retch; sick up; spew; throw up

36. abdomen「腹, 腹部」胸郭と骨盤の間にある体幹の一部。背部の椎骨部は含まないが, 骨盤を含むとする解剖学者もいる。腹腔の大部分を占める。
37. gut「腸」専門用語 intestine の意味で一般的によく使われる。英国の俗語ではお腹, 特に太ったお腹を表す。
38. dyspepsia「消化不良」胃弱, 胃疾患によって起こる胃の機能障害あるいは胃の不調。心窩部の痛み, ときに胃やけ, 吐気, ガス性おくびを特徴とする。
39. oesophagus = esophagus「食道」咽頭から胃までの消化管の部分。

Unit 7　　　　　　　　　　　　　　　　　　　　　　　　　飲食

飲食行動に関連する看護・医学用語あるいは標準英語，並びにそれと対応する口語的な用語と表現が Box. 5 にまとめられている。

注記：病歴と会話例文中における口語的な表現には，〔　〕内に説明を加えた。

BOX. 5

飲食に関連した語

看護・医療用語 または標準的な用語	患者が使う口語的（日常的） または，俗語の（非常にくだけた）用語と表現
腹	腹，消化管〔インフォーマル〕，胃，おなか
腹部痛	腹痛，腹痛〔俗〕，胃痛／おなかの痛み
食欲不振，無食欲，〔拒食症〕	食欲がない
消化不良〔症〕	胃酸過多，胸やけ
食欲旺盛	常時空腹な，もりもり食べる，はらぺこである
口臭	臭い息，口臭
吐き気	胆汁症，吐き気を催す，胃のむかつき
食道	食道〔日常語〕
食欲不振	食べる気になれない，鳥が食べるほども食べない，食事を取らない，空腹でない，食べ物を少しずつ食べる
口内炎	口内潰瘍，口の痛み
嘔吐する	気分が悪くなる，吐く，もどす，食べた物を吐く，〔俗〕吐く，もどす，吐き出す，嘔吐する

Case history 8   Loss of appetite and weight loss: Miss Hyde-Whyte

Miss Hyde-Whyte has come into the community hospital for assessment. She lives alone and has been retired for over 20 years. The district nursing team, who have been visiting Miss Hyde-Whyte to treat her leg ulcer, have recently become concerned about her lack of interest in meals and obvious weight loss.

Nurse: Hello Miss Hyde-Whyte. I'm Nurse Mosquera. I would like to ask you some questions. Will that be all right?

Miss H.: Hello — please call me Maggie. The rest is such a mouthful [difficult to say].

Nurse: I will need to weigh you and measure your height, but first a few questions.

Miss H.: I'm sure that I have lost weight — all my clothes hang on me [are much too big].

Nurse: How often do you eat and drink?

Miss H.: Well I used to have breakfast, a proper cooked lunch and something on toast or a sandwich in the evening.

Nurse: Has something changed?

Miss H.: I used to really enjoy cooking, have a G&T [gin and tonic] and then sit at the table with a nice meal, but now I've got no appetite and I just pick at it [the food]. My dad [father] would have said you don't eat enough to keep a bird alive [have a poor appetite].

Nurse: Why do you think your appetite has decreased?

Miss H.: Two reasons I think. I've had mouth ulcers for ages [a long time]. Probably my false teeth [dentures] don't fit anymore; and I have been sick [vomited] a few times after meals.

Nurse: I'll look at your mouth in a moment [in a short time] and see if any treatment would help. It might be a good idea to

症例8　　食欲不振と体重減：ハイド＝ホワイトさん

ハイド＝ホワイトさんは臨床評価のために地域病院に入院した。彼女は一人暮らしで，退職して20年以上経つ。ハイド＝ホワイトさんの足にできた潰瘍の治療に訪れた地区看護師チームが，彼女の食事への無関心と，明らかな体重の減少について近頃気にかけている。

看護師：　こんにちは，ハイド＝ホワイトさん。看護師のモスクィラーです。少し質問をしたいのですが，よろしいでしょうか？

Hさん：　こんにちは。マギーと呼んでください。後の名前は長すぎます［言うのが難しいです］から。

看護師：　体重と身長を測りますが，まず少し質問をさせてください。

Hさん：　体重は確かに減ったでしょうね。服が全部ぶかぶかです［大きすぎます］。

看護師：　どれくらいの頻度で飲食をしますか？

Hさん：　そうですね，今までは，朝食，ちゃんと料理した昼食，トーストに何かのせたものやサンドイッチを夕食に取っていました。

看護師：　何か変わったことがありましたか。

Hさん：　前は料理がとても好きでした。ジントニ［ジントニック］を飲んで，それからおいしい食べ物を並べてテーブルについていたのです。でも，今はまったく食欲が出なくて，少しだけ［食べ物を］つまむ程度です。私のお父さん［父］なら，「おまえは鳥が食べるほども食べないね［食欲がないね］」と言ったでしょうね。

看護師：　どうして食欲が減退したのだと思いますか？

Hさん：　2つ理由があると思います。ずっと［長い間］口内炎があるんです。きっと入れ歯［義歯］がもう合わないのでしょう。それから，食後に何度か戻した［嘔吐した］ことがあります。

看護師：　口の中をすぐに［間もなく］見てみましょう。どんな治療が役に立つ

25		see your dentist about the poorly fitting dentures. Tell me about the vomiting.
	Miss H.:	If I eat a proper meal I soon feel sick [nauseated] and then I'm sick [vomit]. The food just comes back.
	Nurse:	Are you sick at any other time?
	Miss H.:	No, only after food.
30	Nurse:	What colour is the vomit? Is there any blood or bile?
	Miss H.:	No blood and it's not green or yellow like bile. The colour varies — it depends on what I've eaten.
35	Nurse:	Sometimes blood can look like coffee grounds [describes the appearance of partially digested blood in the vomit] - anything like that?
	Miss H.:	No, nothing like that.
	Nurse:	How do you feel afterwards?
40	Miss H.:	That's the strange thing. Once I've been sick I feel fine [all right]. My stomach [abdomen[36]] feels uncomfortable before I'm sick, but that feeling soon goes afterwards.
	Nurse:	When you were eating normally what sort of food did you cook?
45	Miss H.:	Proper meals — meat or fish and lots of veg. [short for 'vegetables'] and I always had dessert or some cheese. No point doing all that if you're going to be sick.
	Nurse:	How often do you usually shop for food?
	Miss H.:	Most days. It's nice to get out and have a chat [talk] with people.
	Nurse:	What do you eat and drink now?
50	Miss H.:	I know that I must eat something, so I have things like scrambled [a cooking method] egg on toast, soup and milky drinks. It's not unpleasant [In English when you have two negatives, known as a 'double negative', it creates a middle way, meaning 'not a positive' ('a pleasant diet') but
55		not a negative ('an unpleasant diet') either. So here, 'not

(**36. abdomen**「腹, 腹部」)

	か考えます。歯科医に合っていない入れ歯を見てもらうのもいいかもしれません。嘔吐について教えてください。
Hさん：	ちゃんとした食事をするとすぐに気持ちが悪くなって［吐き気がして］，それから戻して［嘔吐して］しまいます。食べ物がただ戻って来てしまうんです。
看護師：	ほかのときは吐き気がしますか？
Hさん：	いいえ，食後だけです。
看護師：	嘔吐物は何色ですか。血液や胆汁は混ざっていますか？
Hさん：	血は混ざっていませんし，胆汁のように緑色でも黄色でもありません。色はさまざまで，何を食べたかによります。
看護師：	血液はコーヒーの出がらしのように見えることがあります［嘔吐物の中に部分的に消化された血液がある様子を説明している］。そのようなことはありませんか？
Hさん：	いいえ，まったくありません。
看護師：	［嘔吐した］後はいかがですか？
Hさん：	それが不思議なんです。戻してしまうと具合が良く［大丈夫に］なります。戻すまでは胃［腹部］が気持ち悪いのですが，［戻した］後はすぐに良くなります。
看護師：	普通に食事をしていたころ，どのようなものを料理していましたか？
Hさん：	ちゃんとした食事です。肉や魚，たくさんの野菜［veg. は vegitable「野菜」の略］です。それから，いつもデザートかチーズを食べていました。吐いてしまうなら何もかも無駄ですけれど。
看護師：	どれくらいの頻度で食品を買いますか？
Hさん：	ほとんど毎日です。外出して，人とおしゃべり［話］をするのは楽しいことです。
看護師：	今はどんなものを食べたり飲んだりしていますか？
Hさん：	何か食べなければいけないのはわかってます。だから，トーストにスクランブルエッグ［卵の調理法の1つ］をのせたものや，スープや乳飲料を取っています。まんざら悪い食事でもないんじゃないでしょうか。［英語で二重否定と呼ばれる，二度否定語を使うときは肯定的な

		unpleasant' means a fairly acceptable diet], but I know it's not enough.
	Nurse:	Let's see how much you weigh. What's your normal weight?
60	Miss H.:	Before the vomiting started I had been about 10 stone [an Imperial Unit of weight where 1 stone = 14 pounds, see Ch. IV] for as long as I can remember [for a long time].
	Nurse:	We use the kilogram for weight, but I can tell what it is in stones and pounds.
65	Miss H.:	What's the verdict [finding] then. Have I lost much?
	Nurse:	I'm afraid [The phrase 'I'm afraid', is used to introduce news which is unwelcome or bad] you have lost about 11kilograms. You weigh 52 kilograms; that's 8 stone 2 pounds, so that's nearly 2 stone less than usual. We will have to keep an eye
70		on [keep a frequent check] your weight.
	Miss H.:	Well, it's no surprise my clothes are much too big.
	Nurse:	I'm going to refer you to the dietician and ask her to come and do a full nutritional assessment and see how we can provide you with enough nutrients and fluid while we wait
75		for all the tests [investigations] to be done. Meanwhile, we can order things like scrambled eggs, and give you soup and drinks with added nutrients [fortified] if you're sure that won't make you sick.
	Miss H.:	I'm sure that will be fine, thank you.

Case history 9   Alcohol abuse: Mr Wakefield

Mr Wakefield is a farmer. His son Tom also works on the farm and lives with his wife and two children in the main farmhouse. Mr Wakefield moved to a smaller house on the farm when his wife died about 6 months ago. The last 6 months have been very difficult for Mr

「良い食事」でも否定的な「悪い食事」でもない，中間の意味を示す。つまりここでは，そこそこ許容範囲内の日常の食事という意味である。〕十分でないことはわかっていますけど。

看護師：　それでは体重を測ってみましょう。普段の体重はどのくらいですか？

Hさん：　嘔吐が始まる前は，覚えている限り〔長い間〕，10ストーン〔英本国法定の重さの単位で1ストーンは14ポンド。第Ⅳ章を参照のこと〕でした。

看護師：　私たちはキログラムを重量の単位として使いますが，ストーンとポンドもわかります。

Hさん：　どうでしたか〔わかりましたか〕。たくさん減っていますか？

看護師：　残念ですが〔'I'm afraid' は歓迎されない，または悪い情報を伝える前に使う表現〕11キロほど体重が落ちています。今52キロで，8ストーン2ポンドですから，普段より2ストーン少ないことになります。体重に注意していかないといけませんね〔頻繁に体重を測る必要があります〕。

Hさん：　服がぶかぶかでしたから，驚きませんね。

看護師：　栄養士に紹介しましょう。彼女に，来てもらって完全な栄養状態の評価を頼みます。検査〔調査〕がすべて終わるのを待つ間に，私たちで充分な栄養と飲み物をどのように〔あなたに〕提供できるか考えてみます。それまでは，スクランブルエッグのようなものを手配できますし，スープと栄養を添加した〔補強した〕飲み物もお出しできます。それで具合が悪くなると思わないなら，ですが。

Hさん：　大丈夫だと思います。ありがとうございます。

症例9　　アルコール乱用：ウェイクフィールド氏

ウェイクフィールドさんは農場主である。息子のトムも同じ農場で働いており，妻と2人の子供と一緒に農場内の母屋に住んでいる。ウェイクフィールドさんは，およそ6か月前に妻が亡くなり，農場の別棟に移った。この6か月はウェイク

Wakefield, and he has come into the health centre to see the practice nurse about feeling generally unwell.

10

Nurse:	Hello Mr Wakefield. How are you today?
Mr W.:	Not up to much [a term used to describe feeling generally unwell or having a low mood]. You know — it's hard to feel interested in anything these days.
Nurse:	Yes, it must be about 6 months since your wife died.
Mr W.:	It will be exactly 6 months on Wednesday. Her dying like that really hit me for six[40] [dealt a severe blow or disappointment]. Tom does his best, but I miss her so much. I can't keep on like this [can't continue in this condition].
Nurse:	What do you mean?
Mr W.:	I can't leave Tom to run [manage] everything, but I feel dreadful [an emotional phrase to express feeling very unwell].
Nurse:	In what way do you feel unwell?
Mr W.:	Most of it's my own fault. I know it's bad for me.
Nurse:	Bad for you?
Mr W.:	The evenings are so long without her [his wife] and at first I thought a couple of drinks [meaning alcoholic drinks] would help me unwind [relax] and get through until bedtime.
Nurse:	Did it help?
Mr W.:	Not really and I ended up having more than a couple of drinks.
Nurse:	Many more?
Mr W.:	Oh yes, most evenings I manage a bottle of wine and some whisky, and then regret it in the morning.
Nurse:	How do you feel in the morning?

40. hit ... for six 「…（人）を打ちのめす」

フィールドさんにとって大変苦しいもので，全般的に気分がすぐれないことについて開業看護師に見てもらうために医療センターに来た。

看護師： こんにちは，ウェイクフィールドさん。今日の気分はいかがですか？

W 氏： そんなにはよくありません［通常具合がよくない場合や気持ちが沈んでいるときに使う表現］。近頃，何事にも興味が持てなくて。

看護師： ええ，奥さまが亡くなられて6か月でしたね。

W 氏： この水曜日でちょうど6か月です。彼女があんな風に死んでしまって，私は打ちのめされました。［深刻な打撃を受けました，がっくりしました］。トムはとてもよくしてくれますが，彼女がいないのが本当にさみしくて。もうこのような状態に耐えられません［この状態を続けられません］。

看護師： どういうことですか？

W 氏： トムにすべてをやらせておくわけにはいきません［切りまわしてもらうわけにはいきません］。でも，本当にひどい気分なのです［とても具合が悪いことを感情的に表現する語句］。

看護師： どのように気分がすぐれないのですか？

W 氏： ほとんどは自分のせいです。よくないことだとはわかっているのですが。

看護師： よくないことというのは？

W 氏： 彼女［彼の妻］のいない夜はとても長く感じられます。最初のうちは，何杯か［お酒を意味する］は，くつろいだり［リラックスしたり］寝るまでの時間をやり過ごすのに役立つと思っていたのです。

看護師： 役に立ちましたか。

W 氏： そうでもありませんでした。結局は 2, 3 杯より多く飲むようになってしまいました。

看護師： もっとたくさんですか？

W 氏： ええ。たいていの晩はワインを1本とウイスキーを少し飲んでしまい，朝になって後悔します。

看護師： 朝はどんな気分ですか？

	Mr W.:	Headache and generally lousy [unwell]. I can't face breakfast and I'm often sick [vomit].
	Nurse:	Do you take anything for the headache?
30	Mr W.:	A couple of aspirin, but they give me terrible [severe] indigestion.
	Nurse:	You have obviously been thinking about the amount of alcohol you drink.
	Mr W.:	Yes, it's worrying me. What if I can't stop and become an alcoholic or something?
35		
	Nurse:	How much do you think you're having in a week?
	Mr W.:	I know that there are sensible limits in units[41], but I don't know what they are.
	Nurse:	Most men can safely drink 3-4 units a day without a significant risk. A unit is 10 grams of alcohol and this is half a pint[42] [an Imperial measure, see Ch. IV] of standard strength beer or one glass of wine or one pub measure of spirits. Some stronger wines have more than I unit. The recommended level is 21-28 units for a man spread over 1 week. It's best to avoid binge drinking [uncontrolled drinking] and keep 1 or 2 days when you don't drink.
40		
45		
	Mr W.:	My intake is well over the sensible limit. Most nights I probably have over 10 units. I need to do something about it.
	Nurse:	You seem to have made up your mind to reduce your intake of alcohol. Have you thought about how you might do this?
50		
	Mr W.:	I don't want to give up [stop] drinking completely. In the past I enjoyed a drink in moderation and that's what I want to aim for. Some people say that they never touch a drop [in this case never drink alcohol], but that's not for me.
55		
	Nurse:	It's good to have a realistic goal, and drinking in

41.unit「ユニット」英国でアルコール摂取量を表す単位。
42.pint「液量単位, パイント」= 1/2 クオート =（米国）28.875 立方インチ = 0.473 リットル =（英国）0.568 リットル = 約 500cc

W 氏： 頭痛がして，だいたい気持ちが悪いです [具合が悪いです]。とても朝食は食べられないし，よく戻します [吐きます]。

看護師： 頭痛に何か飲んでいますか？

W 氏： アスピリンを 2, 3 錠。でもそのせいでひどい [深刻な] 消化不良になります。

看護師： 明らかに飲むお酒の量が気になるようですね。

W 氏： はい，心配です。もしやめられなくてアルコール依存症か何かになったらどうしようかと気になります。

看護師： 1 週間にどのくらい飲んでいると思いますか？

W 氏： アルコールの量に常識的な限度があるのはわかっていますが，それがどれくらいなのかは知りません。

看護師： ほとんどの男性は深刻な危険性なしで 1 日 3 〜 4 ユニットを安全に飲めます。1 ユニットはアルコール 10 グラムで，これは一般の強さのビールを 1 パイントの半分 [pint「パイント」は英本国法定の標準に従った重さの単位。第Ⅳ章を参照] か，グラス 1 杯のワイン，または，パブでのスピリッツ 1 杯にあたります。もっと強いワインは 1 ユニットを超えます。成人男性に推奨できる範囲は，1 週間の間で，21 ユニットから 28 ユニットです。暴飲 [飲みたいだけ飲むの] を避け，1 週間に 1 日か 2 日は飲まない日を設けることも大切です。

W 氏： 私の摂取量は，はるかに良識的な限度を超えています。ほとんど毎晩 10 ユニット以上飲んでいると思います。何とかしなくては。

看護師： アルコール摂取量を減らす決心をしたようですね。どうするか考えたことはありますか？

W 氏： 完全には飲むのをあきらめ [止め] たくはありません。昔は適度にお酒を楽しんでいましたから，またそうなりたいです。1 滴も飲まない [まったく飲まない] という人もいますが，私には当てはまりません。

看護師： 現実的な目標を持つのはいいことです。適度に飲むのは心臓病〔のリ

	moderation may have health benefits, such as reducing heart disease.
Mr W.:	All this booze [slang for alcohol] has made me put on weight [weight increased] so it will be healthier if I cut down [reduce] on drinking and lose weight.
Nurse:	Are evenings the only time that you have a drink?
Mr W.:	Yes, when I'm on my own [alone].
Nurse:	What can you do to change the pattern?
Mr W.:	I used to enjoy a walk round the farm of an evening and my grandsons keep badgering [pestering] me to take them out.
Nurse:	Do you think that's possible?
Mr W.:	Yes, and I think it would help.
Nurse:	I would like to see how you get on [check on your progress]. Perhaps we can make another appointment, and while you're here we can make you an appointment with Doctor Welch. She can arrange for support from a counsellor, and she might think that you would benefit from some medication.
Mr W.:	Yes, I know I need some proper help and it's such a relief to have told someone about my drinking. I could never tell Tom. It would cause too much bother [upset].

	スク〕を減らすなど，健康に良い可能性があります。
W氏：	この酒［boozeはアルコールの俗語］のせいで太った［体重が増えた］のですから，飲酒量を少なくして［減らして］やせたら健康的ですね。
看護師：	お酒を飲むのは夜だけですか？
W氏：	そうです，私だけ［1人だけ］のときです。
看護師：	習慣を変えるのに何ができると思いますか？
W氏：	以前は，夕方農場を散歩するのが好きでした。孫たちが連れていってほしいとせがんだ［しつこかった］ものです。
看護師：	〔また〕できると思いますか？
W氏：	はい，助けになると思います。
看護師：	どうやっていくか見たい［経過をチェックしたい］と思います。次の予約を取りましょうか，そしてここにいる間に，ウェルチ先生の予約もできます。彼女はカウンセラーの支援を手配してくれますし，投薬が効果的か検討するかもしれませんね。
W氏：	ええ，私にはちゃんとした助けが必要だとわかっています。お酒のことを人に話せて本当によかったです。トムには決して言えません。騒ぎになって［心配させて］しまうでしょうから。

Unit 8   ELIMINATION

Some nursing/medical or Standard English words and corresponding colloquial words and expressions associated with elimination are given in Box. 6.

Note: Colloquial expressions used in the case histories and example conversations are explained in brackets […].

BOX. 6
Words associated with elimination

Nursing/medical or Standard English words	Colloquial (everyday) or slang (very informal) words and expressions used by patients
Constipation	Bunged up; clogged up; costive; haven't been for days; not going properly
Defaecate	Go to the toilet; have bowels open; do number two; pass a motion or stool; to do one's business; to have a clear out
Diarrhoea	Gippy tummy; loose motion; runs; squitters; to be taken short; trots
Faeces; stool	Business; motion; number two; pooh
Flatulence	Belching; feel bloated; gas; wind
Incontinence[43]	Have an accident; I leak; leaky; messed myself; not able to hold on; wet myself
Micturition/urinate	Number one; go to the loo/toilet; pass water[44]; pass urine. pee; spend a penny; tiddle; wee or wee-wee

---

43. incontinence「失禁」incontinence は失禁と訳されるが, in- は否定を意味する接頭辞で, continence「コンチネンス」でない状態が incontinence である。continence は「禁制」と訳されてきたが, 単語の持つ意味を表すには十分でなく「コンチネンス」と訳しておくのがよいと考える。コンチネンスは, 排泄〔尿・便〕がコントロールできている状態を表す。
44. pass water「お小水をする」

Unit 8　　　　　　　　　　　　　　　　　　　　　排泄

排泄に関連する看護・医学用語あるいは標準英語，並びにそれと対応する口語的な用語と表現が Box. 6 にまとめられている。

注記：病歴と会話例文中における口語的な表現には，〔　〕内に説明を加えた。

BOX. 6

排泄に関連した語

看護・医療用語 または標準的な用語	患者が使う口語的（日常的） または，俗語の（非常にくだけた）用語と表現
便秘	詰まった，詰まった，便秘を起こさせる，何日もない，ちゃんとしていない
排便する	トイレに行く，お通じをする，大きいほうをする，排便する，おつとめをする，すっきりする
下痢	〔特に旅行者がかかる〕下痢，ゆるい便，下痢，〔俗〕下痢，急に〔トイレに〕行きたくなる，〔俗語〕下痢になること
糞便・大便	おつとめ，便通，大きいほう，うんち
鼓腸	少量のガスを出すこと，膨張感がする，ガス，おなら
〔大小便の〕失禁	お漏らしをする，漏らす，汚す，我慢できない，濡らす
排尿・排尿する	小さいほう，トイレに行く，小水をする，排尿をする，〔幼児語〕おしっこ，〔英話〕トイレに行く，小便，〔幼児語〕おしっこをする

Lavatory	Bathroom; bog; cloakroom; convenience; gents'; ladies'; latrine; lav.; little girls' room; 100; privy; smallest room; toilet; washroom; water closet (WC)
Urine	Pee; water
Urinary tract	Waterworks[45] (especially the bladder)

Case history 10   Urinary incontinence: Mrs Carter

Mrs Carter has been admitted to the coronary care unit[46] for treatment of unstable angina[47]. She has had angina for about 2 years. During a conversation about the need to use a commode[48] by the bed in order to reduce exertion and hence the oxygen needed by the heart muscle
5 [myocardium], she tells you that she has trouble with her waterworks [urinary tract, especially the bladder].

🔘 11

Nurse: What sort of problem with your waterworks?
Mrs C.: I can't hold on and I leak urine [incontinent of urine]. It's so embarrassing.
Nurse: It sounds like you have two separate problems.
5 Mrs C.: I hadn't thought of it as two problems, but it does happen at different times. The main problem is the need to pass water [micturate] so often and when I need the toilet [lavatory] it is all of a rush [urgent]. Sometimes I don't make it in time and wet myself [incontinent of urine]. The leaking happens
10   when I cough or laugh.
Nurse: How often do you pass water [micturate]?

---
45. water works「泌尿器」英口語
46. coronary care unit「冠疾患集中治療室」略語は CCU。
47. angina「狭心症」angina pectoris とも。
48. commode「室内用便器」(特に病人用の) 椅子型ポータブル便器。

洗面所〔トイレ〕	バスルーム,〔俗〕トイレ,〔英〕トイレ,お手洗い,〔英俗〕男性用公衆トイレ,女性用公衆トイレ,〔キャンプ地などの公衆の〕トイレ,トイレ〔lavatory の婉曲語〕,〔英話〕おトイレ,トイレ,個室,小部屋,トイレ,お手洗い,トイレ(WC)
尿	おしっこ,小水
尿路	泌尿器系(特に膀胱)

症例 10　コンチネンス・ケア(尿失禁のケア):カーター夫人

カーター夫人は,不安定狭心症の治療のために冠疾患集中治療室に入院している。彼女は約 2 年間狭心症を患っている。激しい運動の量を減らし,心臓の筋肉[心筋]の酸素必要量を減らすため,ベッドのそばの室内用便器を使う必要があることについて話している間,彼女は泌尿器系[尿管,特に膀胱]に問題があることを話す。

看護師:　排尿についてどんな問題がありますか?
C 夫人:　お小水を我慢することができなくて,漏らしてしまいます[尿失禁です]。とても恥ずかしいです。
看護師:　どうも 2 つの別々の問題があるようですね。
C 夫人:　2 つの問題だととらえていませんでしたが,確かに起こるのは別々のときです。おもな問題は,お小水[排尿]が非常に頻繁なのと,急に[緊急に]トイレ[洗面所]に行きたくなることです。間に合わなくて漏らしてしまうこと[尿失禁]もあります。咳をしたり,笑ったりしても漏れます。
看護師:　何度くらいお小水[排尿]をしますか?

Mrs C.:	Every couple [two] of hours or so [approximately] during the day.
Nurse:	What about at night, do you have to get up in the night [to pass water]?
Mrs C.:	Oh yes, I have to keep getting up [frequently get out of bed to urinate]. Always twice a night and sometimes more often.
Nurse:	When did you start having problems?
Mrs C.:	Just after I retired. I'm 68 now, so it must be about 4 years ago.
Nurse:	Have you told your GP or the practice nurse?
Mrs C.:	I felt too embarrassed and it's something that happens when you get older isn't it? It really limits my social life and it worries me that I might smell.
Nurse:	It is more common in older people, but there are different causes and many can be successfully treated. How do you normally cope with the problem?
Mrs C.:	I try to be near a toilet, but that's not always easy if I'm out. There are not many public toilets and some of them are not very clean. I wear a sanitary towel [normally used during menstruation] in my knickers [pants, underwear] to cope with the leaks, but I still have plenty of washing to do [implying that this does not always work].
Nurse:	I will add all this to your care plan and make sure that everyone knows to bring the commode as soon as you ask. Would you like a supply of towels and disposal bags to keep in the locker?
Mrs C.:	Yes please.
Nurse:	When your angina has settled down and you are feeling better I will arrange for the continence nurse specialist to come to see you. She is the expert and will be able to do a full assessment and suggest ways of improving the situation.
Mrs C.:	I wish I'd told someone earlier, but I thought that you had to

C夫人：	日中は2,3時間[2]時間ぐらい[おおよそ]ごとです。
看護師：	夜間はいかがですか。夜中に[排尿のため]に起きなければなりませんか？
C夫人：	はい，何度も起きなければ[排尿のために頻繁にベッドを出なければ]なりません。いつもはだいたい2回で，もっと多いこともあります。
看護師：	いつから問題が始まりましたか？
C夫人：	ちょうど退職後からです。今68歳ですから，約4年前でしょう。
看護師：	今までにかかりつけ医か開業看護師に話したことはありますか？
C夫人：	恥ずかしすぎましたし，こういうことは年をとると起こるでしょう？社会生活はとても制限されますし，臭うのではと心配になります。
看護師：	お年寄りに多いですが，原因はさまざまですし，多くの人は治療がうまくいきます。普段はどういう風に対処していますか？
C夫人：	トイレの近くにいるようにしています。外出しているときにはなかなかそうはいきませんけど。公衆トイレがたくさんあるわけではないし，あまりきれいでないところもあります。ナプキン[普通は生理中に使用されるもの]をパンティ[パンティ，下着]に付けて，漏れに対処しています。それでも洗い物がたくさんあります[この方法ではうまくいっていないことを暗示している]。
看護師：	このことは看護計画にすべて書き加えておきます。そしてみんなに，頼まれたらすぐに室内用便器を持って来るよう伝えます。ナプキンや使い捨ての袋をロッカーに入れておきましょうか？
C夫人：	お願いします。
看護師：	狭心症が落ち着いて具合がよくなったらコンチネンス・ケア〔尿失禁のケア〕を専門にしている看護師士の予約を手配しましょう。彼女は専門家で，すべての検査をして，状況が良くなるようアドバイスしてくれます。
C夫人：	もっと早くだれかにお話すればよかったのですが，笑って耐えなけれ

45		grin and bear it [put up with it]. I had no idea that anything could be done.
	Nurse:	While we're waiting I'd like to have a specimen [sample] of your water to test, and if that shows that you might have an infection we can collect a midstream specimen of urine for the laboratory.
50	Mrs C.:	Is that the test where you have to pee [micturate] into a pot?
	Nurse:	Yes, that's the one, but we only need the middle bit of the flow, not the urine that comes out first. Have you noticed any blood in your urine or an unusual smell?
	Mrs C.:	No, nothing like that.
55	Nurse:	What about pain when you pass urine? Does it burn or sting?
	Mrs C.:	No, I had cystitis[49] when I was younger and I know how painful it is when you go[50] [when she passes urine; micturates].
60	Nurse:	We also need to know how often you are passing urine and how much fluid you are having, but as we are already recording fluid balance for you we will have that information.
	Mrs C.:	You will tell the nurses about how urgent it is when I ask for the commode?
65	Nurse:	Don't worry I'm putting it on the care plan now, and I will tell the nurse who takes over from me tonight. Do you think you could give me that sample now?
	Mrs C.:	Yes.
70	Nurse:	Have you any questions before I go and get the commode?
	Mrs C.:	No, I'm looking forward to feeling better and seeing the specialist nurse about the waterworks.

49.cystitis「膀胱炎」
50.(when) you go「トイレに行く, 排尿する(とき)」

ばならない［我慢しなければならない］ことだと思っていました。何かできるなんて思いもよりませんでした。

看護師： 待っている間に，検査のための尿の試料［サンプル］を取りたいのですが。もし感染症の疑いがあると出たら，臨床検査のために中間尿を採取することになります。

C夫人： ポットしびんにお小水［排尿］をしなければならない検査ですか？

看護師： ええ，それです。でも必要なのは，初尿ではなく，尿流の中のほんの少しの中間尿です。尿に血液が混じっていたり，異臭がしたことに気がついたことはありますか？

C夫人： いいえ，そのようなことはありません。

看護師： 排尿のときに痛みはありますか？焼けるような痛みや刺すような痛みは？

C夫人： いいえ，若いときに膀胱炎になったことがありますから，トイレに行く［尿を出す，排尿する］ときにどんなに痛いかは知っています。

看護師： どのくらいの頻度で排尿するか，どのくらい水分を取っているかを知る必要もあります。でも，すでに水分バランスを記録してありますから，そのデータは得られるでしょう。

C夫人： 私が頼むときは，どんなに差し迫って室内用便器が必要か，看護師さんたちに話してくださいね？

看護師： 大丈夫ですよ，今，看護計画にそのことを書き加えているところです。それから，今夜私の後を引き継ぐ看護師に伝えます。今，検体を出せると思いますか？

C夫人： はい。

看護師： 室内用便器を取りに行く前に何か質問はありますか？

C夫人： いいえ，気分が良くなって泌尿器についての専門看護師に会うのが楽しみです。

Case history 11   Constipation: Mr Norton

Mr Norton fractured his femur[51] in a motorcycle accident 2 weeks ago. The fracture is being managed with skeletal traction[52] and Mr Norton has accepted that he will be much less active than usual and will be in hospital for some weeks. He had started to feel better after the accident and the pain in his leg was gradually subsiding, but now he feels bloated [blown up, distended], lethargic and has no appetite.

Mr N.:   I feel terrible [very bad], really out of sorts [unwell].
Nurse: What's the trouble?
Mr N.:   I haven't been properly for days [has not defaecated properly for days and is constipated].
Nurse: When did you last have your bowels open [defaecate]?
Mr N.:   Saturday was OK, so that's 4 days ago. I wish I'd said earlier, but it seemed stupid to be worried about not going [defaecating] when I'm laid-up [confined to bed] with a leg that's broke [fractured].
Nurse: How often do you usually go?
Mr N.:   Every day without fail.
Nurse: It's probably happened because you're not as active as usual and having to use a bedpan[53] doesn't help.
Mr N.:   Well I can't do much with the traction and stuff.
Nurse: How is it making you feel?
Mr N.:   I'm all blown up and full of wind [flatulence]. Look at my stomach [abdomen], it's huge. I couldn't eat nothing[54] and my mum [mother] had brought in a Chinese [a

---

51. femur　「大腿骨」
52. skeletal traction　「直達牽引」長骨の骨折を整復するために、骨に差し込んだ金属釘や鋼線で骨を牽引する。
53. bedpan　「ベッドパン」寝たきりの患者が使う便器。差し込み便器とも。
54. I couldn't eat nothing　「私は何も食べられない」否定語が2度用いられているが、ここでは否定を表す。会話ではこのような不正確な文章も使われることがある。

症例11　　便秘：ノートン氏

ノートン氏は，2週間前にオートバイの事故により大腿骨を骨折した。骨折は直達牽引で治療されており，彼はいつもよりずっと活動性が鈍くなってしまうことや，数週間入院することを受け入れている。事故の後，具合が次第に良くなり脚の痛みも徐々に治まってきた。しかし，現在は〔腹部が〕膨張した感じがして〔膨れ上がっている，膨張感がある〕，無気力で食欲がない。

N氏：　　すごく体調が悪い〔具合が悪い〕です。本当に元気が出ません〔体調がすぐれません〕。

看護師：　どうしました？

N氏：　　何日も〔便が〕出ないんです〔きちんと排便がなく，便秘である〕。

看護師：　最後に便が出た〔排便があった〕のはいつですか。

N氏：　　土曜日は大丈夫でした。だから4日前ですね。もっと早く言えばよかったんですが，脚の骨を折って〔骨折して〕ベッドで寝ている〔病床にある〕ときに，出ないこと〔排便〕を心配するなんてばかばかしい気がして。

看護師：　いつもはどのくらいの頻度で出ますか？

N氏：　　間違いなく毎日です。

看護師：　いつもほど体を動かさないからだと思います。病人用のベッドパンを使わなければならないのは楽ではないですし。

N氏：　　牽引なんかしていると自由が利きません。

看護師：　出ないせいでどんな感じがしますか？

N氏：　　ものすごく膨満感があって，ガスがたまっている感じ〔鼓腸感〕がします。腹〔腹部〕を見てみてください。巨大ですよ。まったく何も食べられないので，母さん〔母〕が特別に中華〔テイクアウトの食事〕を持ってきてくれました。

		takeaway[55] meal] as a treat.
20	Nurse:	Yes, your abdomen is a bit distended. Have you any pain?
	Mr N.:	A bit. It feels like colic[56] [usually refers to intermittent abdominal pain, most often from the intestine, but sometimes from other structures].
	Nurse:	What was your motion[57] [faeces; stool] like on Saturday?
25	Mr N.:	Just a few hard bits and I had to strain [push hard] to get that out.
	Nurse:	What it's like normally?
	Mr N.:	Normal — soft and not having to strain. Except when I've got the runs [diarrhea] after too much beer and a curry.
30	Nurse:	Was there any pain passing the hard motion, or blood when you cleaned yourself?
	Mr N.:	No pain and I didn't see no blood. If I had I would have said straight away [immediately, at once].
	Nurse:	Did you feel that you hadn't passed a complete motion?
35	Mr N.:	Yeah [yes], my back passage [rectum] felt full just as if there was more to come.
	Nurse:	I'll get Dr Cox to write you up for [prescribe] some medicine [laxative] to make you go and we can ask the physio. [short for 'physiotherapist'] to suggest some exercises to help.
40	Mr N.:	My gran [grandmother] swears by [relies on] her bottle of bowel medicine.
	Nurse:	You might need some suppositories or a micro enema to get things started and then a few doses of an oral laxative. Hopefully you won't need a whole bottle. It will also help
45		if you can drink more water and choose food high in fibre from the menu.
	Mr N.:	Yeah alright, but I don't want salad every meal.

---

55. takeaway「テイクアウト」米口語では takeout だが, 英口語では takeaway と表現することが多い。
56. colic「疝痛」腹部のけいれん痛を表す。
57. motion「排便, 便通, 通じ」

看護師：	そうですね，腹部が少し張ってますね。痛みはありますか？
N氏：	少し。差し込みみたいな痛み［通常，間欠性の腹部の痛みを言い，多くの場合は腸から来る痛みであるが，ほかが原因の場合もある］です。
看護師：	土曜日に出たの［排泄物，便］はどんなでしたか。
N氏：	とても硬い小さいのがいくつかだけで，出すのにかなり力を入れなければ［力まなければ］なりませんでした。
看護師：	普段はどうですか？
N氏：	普通です。軟らかくて，力を入れなくても平気です。ビールを飲み過ぎてカレーを食べた後に下痢になったときを除いて。
看護師：	硬い排便のときは痛みますか。または，拭いたときに血が付いたことは？
N氏：	痛みはないし，血もまったく見てません。もし見ていたらすぐ［即時に，すぐさま］に言ってますよ。
看護師：	排便が完全に終わっていない感じはありましたか？
N氏：	まあ［はい］。お尻の奥［直腸］あたりに，まだ出てくるような，詰まっているような感じがありました。
看護師：	コックス先生に〔便が〕出るようになる薬［下剤］を出して［処方して］もらいましょう。それから physio［physio. は physiotherapist「理学療法士」の略］に役立つ運動を提案してもらいましょう。
N氏：	おばあちゃん［祖母］は彼女の1瓶の腸薬が絶対効くと信じて［頼って］ました。
看護師：	便通を促すのに座薬か小さい浣腸が必要になるかもしれません。それから経口の下剤数錠も。1瓶まるごとはいらないと思いますけど。もっとたくさん水を飲んだり，メニューから食物繊維の多い食べ物を選ぶのも役に立ちます。
N氏：	ええ，わかりました。でも，毎回の食事にサラダは嫌ですよ。

Unit 9 PERSONAL CARE — CLEANSING AND DRESSING, SKIN CARE

Some nursing/medical or Standard English words and corresponding colloquial words and expressions associated with personal care are given in Box. 7.

Note: Colloquial expressions used in the case histories and example conversations are explained in brackets [...].

BOX. 7
Words associated with personal care

Nursing/medical or Standard English words	Colloquial (everyday) or slang (very informal) words and expressions used by patients
Bath/bathe	Have a soak; scrub down
Contusion	Bruise
Dandruff	Scurf
Emollient	Moisturiser
Erythema	Redness
Excoriation	Soreness
Halitosis	Bad breath; mouth odour
Oral hygiene	Brush/clean teeth; mouth wash
Pressure ulcer	Bedsore; pressure sore
Pruritus	Itching (intense)
Rash	Spots/spotty
Wash	Hair wash; hands and face wash; strip wash; wash at the sink/basin

Unit 9　日常生活の介護 ― 洗浄と身支度，スキンケア

　日常生活の介護に関連する看護・医学用語あるいは標準英語，並びにそれと対応する口語的な用語と表現が Box. 7 にまとめられている。

注記：病歴と会話例文中における口語的な表現には，〔　〕内に説明を加えた。

BOX. 7

日常生活の介護に関連した語

看護・医療用語 または標準的な用語	患者が使う口語的（日常的） または，俗語の（非常にくだけた）用語と表現
入浴，入浴させる	〔風呂・水に〕浸かる，ゴシゴシ洗う〔こする〕
挫傷〔打撲傷〕	打ち身〔あざ〕
ふけ症	ふけ
緩和薬〔皮膚軟化薬〕	保湿剤
紅斑	赤み
すり傷〔瘡痕〕	〔ひりひりする〕痛み
口臭	臭い息，口臭
口腔衛生	歯を磨く / 歯を磨く，うがい薬
褥瘡性潰瘍	床ずれ，褥瘡
そう痒	かゆみ（強烈な）
発疹〔皮疹〕	吹き出物，にきびがある
洗浄〔液〕	洗髪液，ハンドソープ・洗顔料，〔裸になって〕体を洗う，洗面台・洗面器で洗う

Case history 12   Geriatric deterioration: Mrs McBride

Mrs McBride lives alone, and Sue her daughter-in-law [the wife of Mrs McBride's son] pops in [visits] most days to take her a meal and check that she is all right. Recently, Sue has noticed that Mrs McBride is increasingly frail[58] and takes a long time to answer the door or make a drink.

🔘 13

Nurse: Hello Mrs McBride. I'm Nurse Ramos. I think you are expecting me. I've come in to see how you are managing at home.

Mrs M.: Hello dear [an endearment often used by older people] come in. Yes, I knew you were coming. Sue mentioned it earlier when she was in with my lunch [meal in the middle of the day]. She's a good girl to me.

Nurse: I've got a checklist to complete, but it's usually better if you tell me in your own words how you think you are managing. What about if we start with any difficulties you might be having with washing and dressing?

Mrs M.: Yes, that's fine. I've always been as fit as a fiddle[59] [in very good health], but since the winter it's got more and more difficult. Well I am 83. It's all down to [as a result of] old age I suppose.

Nurse: What's more difficult?

Mrs M.: I struggle a bit with a strip wash [wash all over] at the sink, but I get by [cope]. My feet and back don't get done, and it's hard to stand up to wash down below [genital and perianal area]. I need to hold on to[60] the sink and then I can't soap the flannel.

---
58. frail「虚弱な」
59. as fit as a fiddle「とても元気［健康］である」語源は fiddle「バイオリンの弦」がピンと張っている様子とされる。
60. hold on to ...「～にしっかりしがみつく」

症例12　加齢による機能低下：マックブライド夫人

マックブライド夫人は1人住まいで，スーという義理の娘［マックブライド夫人の息子の嫁］がほぼ毎日彼女のところに立ち寄り［を訪ね］，食事を運んだり様子を見たりしている。最近，スーはマックブライド夫人がだんだん体が弱くなってきていて，玄関に出てきたり，飲み物を作るのに時間がかかることに気がついた。

看護師：　こんにちは，マックブライドさん。看護師のラモスです。訪問についてはご存じでしょう。家での生活をどのようにやりくりしているか見に来ました。

M夫人：　こんにちは，看護師さん［dear は年配の人が使う，親愛を込めた相手への呼びかけ］。お入りください。ええ，いらっしゃることは知っていました。スーが昼食［お昼に食べる食事］を持って来たときに話していました。彼女はとてもよくしてくれています。

看護師：　記入するためのチェックリストを持ってきていますが，だいたいの場合は，ご自身の言葉で，やっていることについてどう思っているか話してもらうほうがいいです。体を洗うことや，身支度で困っていることから始めるのはどうでしょう。

M夫人：　ええ，いいですよ。私はいつでも体の調子が良かったのです［とても健康でした］が，この冬からどんどんつらくなってきています。そう，83歳ですから，みんな年をとったせい［ことが原因］でしょうね。

看護師：　どんなことがつらくなりましたか？

M夫人：　流しで身体を洗う［身体中を洗う］のが大変です。どうにかしています［対処しています］けど。足や背中は洗えませんし，下の方［性器や肛門付近］を洗うのに立ち上がりづらいです。洗面台にしっかりしがみつかなければならず，そうすると石鹸で〔浴用の〕タオルフランネルを泡立てられません。

Nurse:	Are you able to have a bath or shower?
Mrs M.:	No, I'm not strong enough to get in and out of the bath. I'm frightened of slipping, or getting in and not getting out again.
Nurse:	How often did you have a bath when you were able to manage?
Mrs M.:	Two or three times a week. Heating the water with the immersion heater[61] costs too much to have a bath every day.
Nurse:	How do you heat the water for your strip wash?
Mrs M.:	Boil a kettle; I've got one in the bedroom for a cuppa[62] [usually refers to a cup of tea] in the morning. Would you like a cup of tea now?
Nurse:	No thanks I had one [cup of tea] just before I came out to see you. Would you like to have a bath if it was possible?
Mrs M.:	Oh yes, there's nothing like a soak in the bath for getting clean and relaxing you.
Nurse:	I quite agree. Is there anyone who could help you?
Mrs M.:	I can't ask Sue. She has three children to get off to school, and I don't want to sit in my dressing gown[63] until she can get here.
Nurse:	Would you consider having a bath seat[64] that lowers you into the bath and then goes up when you're ready to get out?
Mrs M.:	I'm hopeless with machines. How easy are they to use?
Nurse:	Very easy. You have a button to push that lowers and raises the seat. If you like we can arrange for someone

---

61. immersion heater 「ロッド式湯沸かし電熱器」水に器具を浸し加熱してお湯を沸かす。
62. cuppa 「〔英・豪口語〕1杯の紅茶・お茶・コーヒー」cup of tea [coffee] の cup of を縮めた発音から。
63. dressing gown 「部屋着」長くゆったりした衣類。パジャマなどの上にはおる。米語 bathrobe 「バスローブ、〔ナイト〕ガウン」と同様の意味を持つ。
64. bath seat 「入浴補助リフト」電動のリフト機能を備える椅子型の簡単な装置。入浴を補助する。

看護師：　入浴したり，シャワーを浴びることはできますか？

M夫人：　できません。バスタブに入ってまた出るほど体力がありません。滑ったり，〔バスタブの〕中に入って出られなくなるのが怖いんです。

看護師：　どうにかできていたころは，どのくらいの頻度で入浴してましたか？

M夫人：　1週間に2，3回です。入浴を毎日するには，ロッド式湯わかし電熱器でお湯を沸かすのは費用がかさみ過ぎます。

看護師：　身体を洗うお湯はどうやって沸かしていますか？

M夫人：　やかんで沸かします。朝1杯［普通は1杯のお茶を指す］飲むために寝室にやかんを置いています。今，お茶を1杯いかがですか？

看護師：　いいえ結構です。会いに来る直前に1杯［お茶を］飲んできましたから。もし可能なら入浴したいですか？

M夫人：　ええ，もちろんです。体をきれいにしてリラックスするには，お風呂に浸かるのが1番ですから。

看護師：　本当にそうですね。どなたか補助してくれる人はいらっしゃいますか？

M夫人：　スーには頼めません。彼女は3人の子供を学校に送り出さなければならないし，私も彼女が来るまで部屋着のままで待ちたくありません。

看護師：　入浴補助リフトの設置を考えてみてはいかがですか？〔シートに座ったまま〕お風呂の中に下げることができて，出たくなったら上げればいいのです。

M夫人：　機械はまったく苦手なのですよ。どのくらい簡単に使えますか？

看護師：　とても簡単です。シートを下したり上げたりするのに押すボタンがあ

50 Mrs M.:	from Social Services[65] to come out and do an assessment. What about washing your hair? That's no problem. I can do it at the sink. My neighbour used to be a hairdresser and she comes in every few weeks and gives it a cut and set.
Nurse:	That's handy [convenient].
Mrs M.:	It certainly is. I can't get down the town these days unless Sue takes me. I haven't been shopping on my own for ages [for a long time].
Nurse:	Do you have any problems getting dressed and undressed?
Mrs M.:	Some things take for ever [a long time], like putting on tights or trousers.
Nurse:	What about doing things up - buttons and zips, etc.?
Mrs M.:	I make sure that clothes do up[66] at the front - no good struggling with a zip at the back of a dress.
Nurse:	The occupational therapist can suggest some simple gadgets [appliances, devices] to help with dressing and show you about easier ways of doing things. Would you like me to arrange for her to come?
Mrs M.:	Yes please. Another neighbour, Mrs Smith at number 80 [the house number], had a visit from one of them and she got on very well.

Case history 13   Eczema: Mr Dafnis

Mr Dafnis is going to have planned [elective] surgery. He has a long history of eczema, with dry, itchy skin. When he attends the pre-admission assessment clinic he expresses some concern about the care of his skin condition while he is in the ward after the major surgical operation.

65. Social Service 〔英〕通常は政府の「社会福祉団体」
66. do up「〔衣服のボタンを〕留める, かける」

	るのです。もしよろしかったら，社会福祉団体からだれかに来て調べてもらうよう手配できます。洗髪はどうなさっていますか？
M夫人：	まったく問題ありません。洗面台でできます。近所の方で以前美容師をしてた人がいて，2, 3週間に1度来てカットとセットをしてくれるのですよ。
看護師：	それは重宝［便利］ですね。
M夫人：	本当にそうなのです。このごろはスーが連れて行ってくれなければ町にも行けません。もうずっと［長い間］1人で買い物に行っていません。
看護師：	服を着たり脱いだりするのは大変ではありませんか？
M夫人：	永遠に［長い間］時間がかかることもあります。タイツを履いたり，ズボンを履いたりといったことなんかは。
看護師：	ボタンやチャックなどを留めることはどうですか？
M夫人：	必ず前で留める服にしています。服の後ろに付いているチャックで苦労するなんて無駄ですから。
看護師：	作業療法士が，身支度を補助する簡単で気の利いた小物［機器，装置］や，いろいろなことをするとき楽な方法を教えてくれます。彼女が来るよう手配しましょうか？
M夫人：	はい，お願いします。別の近所の人で，80番［家の番地］に住んでいるスミスさんも作業療法士さんに来てもらって，とてもうまくやっています。

症例13　　湿疹：ダフニス氏

ダフニスさんは予定の［待機］手術を受けることになっている。彼は長い間痒みのある乾燥肌で，湿疹を患っている。術前検査外来に来ていて，大きな外科手術の後に病棟で過ごす間の皮膚の手入れについて懸念を示している。

Mr D.:	I'm worried about my eczema when I come into hospital. It's important to follow my usual routine or it will flare up[67] [get worse] again.
Nurse:	How long have you had eczema?
Mr D.:	For years, it's chronic now but some things make it worse.
Nurse:	What sort of things?
Mr D.:	In my case it's things like getting too hot, such as from the sun shining through a window.
Nurse:	We can arrange for you to have a bed well away from any windows. Is there anything else?
Mr D.:	Alcohol starts up the itching [pruritus], but I never touch it [does not drink alcohol] nowadays.
Nurse:	What's your skin like now?
Mr D.:	Not very good. It's very red [erythema] and the itching and scratching is much worse. I put it down to [caused by] the stress of having to have the op. [short for 'operation'].
Nurse:	Which areas are worse affected?
Mr D.:	Mainly my face, as you can see, and my back is very itchy.
Nurse:	Have you any sore areas [excoriation] or weeping [producing exudate] areas?
Mr D.:	No, my skin is just dry and very itchy. Any vesicles[68] and broken areas would mean I was open to infection. Is that why you're asking?
Nurse:	Yes, exactly. But to be on the safe side[69] I'll get the doctor to have a look now. What measures are you taking to reduce the flare up?
Mr D.:	I never use soap because it takes out my natural skin oils, so I use soap substitute, and at the moment I'm using an oily

67. flare up「急に悪くなる」
68. vesicle「小疱, 小水疱, 小発疹」
69. to be on the safe side「念のために, 大事をとるなら」

D 氏 : 入院するとき,湿疹が〔どうなるのか〕心配です。いつも同じように手当することは重要で,そうしないとまた急に悪くなる［悪化する］でしょう。

看護師 : 湿疹が出てからどのくらいになりますか？

D 氏 : もう何年も経ちます。今では慢性になってしまいましたが,何かの拍子に悪くなります。

看護師 : どのようなことですか？

D 氏 : 私の場合,暑くなりすぎるようなことです。例えば,窓から入る日光のせいで。

看護師 : どの窓からもちゃんと離れた位置にあるベッドを手配しますよ。ほかにはありますか？

D 氏 : アルコールで痒く［そう痒に］なります。でも近頃はまったく飲みません［お酒を飲みません］。

看護師 : 今は皮膚の具合はどうですか？

D 氏 : あまり良くありません。とても赤くて［紅斑であり］,痒みも,ひっかき傷ももっとひどくなっています。オペ［op. は operation「手術」の略］を受けなければならないストレスから来ている［が原因］と思います。

看護師 : どこが悪くなっていますか？

D 氏 : ご覧になっておわかりのように,主に顔です。それに背中もとても痒いです。

看護師 : ヒリヒリする［皮膚剥脱の］ところやジクジクする［滲出液が出る］ところはありますか？

D 氏 : いえ,皮膚が乾燥して痒いだけです。小水泡や傷ついたところがあると,感染しやすいということですよね。それが質問の意図ですか？

看護師 : ええ,その通りです。でも念のため,すぐお医者さんに見てもらうようにします。突然悪くならないようにどんな方法を取っていますか？

D 氏 : 皮膚にもともとある油脂を取ってしまうので,絶対に石鹸を使わないで,代用物を使っています。それから,今は油分の多い保湿液［軟化

30		moisturiser [emollient] nearly every hour, but touch wood [a reference to the habit of touching something wooden to avert bad luck] it won't be so bad by the time I come into the ward.
	Nurse:	Are you using anything other than the emollient on your skin?
35	Mr D.:	No.
	Nurse:	Have you used steroid ointments lately?
	Mr D.:	No, not for months. I only have them as a last resort[70].
	Nurse:	What about other medicines?
	Mr D.:	I'm taking an antihistamine so the scratching is reduced and
40		I can get some sleep.
	Nurse:	I'll make sure that your skin management is written in the care plan. Have you any questions?
	Mr D.:	What if my eczema gets really bad before I'm due to come in?
	Nurse:	If it gets any worse please let us know. I'll be giving you
45		some printed information with the unit telephone number in any case.
	Mr D.:	OK, thanks.

70. last resort「最後の手段」

薬] をほとんど1時間ごとに塗っています。病棟に入るまでにそんなに悪くなりませんように [touch wood は悪運を避けるために木製のものに touch する慣習から，おまじないのように使われる]。

看護師： 軟化薬の他に皮膚に何か使用していますか？

D氏： いいえ。

看護師： 最近ステロイドの軟膏は使いましたか？

D氏： いいえ，何か月もないです。最後の手段として持っているだけです。

看護師： 他の薬はいかがですか？

D氏： なるべく掻かないように抗ヒスタミン剤を飲んでいます。それで少し眠れますから。

看護師： 看護計画に皮膚管理について必ず書くようにします。何か質問はありますか？

D氏： 入院予定日の前に湿疹がひどく悪くなったらどうしたらいいでしょう？

看護師： もし今より悪くなったら教えてください。いずれにせよ，病棟の電話番号が載っている資料をお渡ししますね。

D氏： はい，ありがとうございます。

Unit 10 SLEEPING

Some nursing/medical or Standard English words and corresponding colloquial words and expressions associated with sleeping are given in Box. 8.

Note: Colloquial expressions used in the case histories and example conversations are explained in brackets [...].

BOX. 8

Words associated with sleeping

Nursing/medical or Standard English words	Colloquial (everyday) or slang (very informal) words and expressions used by patients
Bruxism	Grind my teeth during sleep
Go to bed/sleep	Hit the hay/sack[71]; retire for the night; say goodnight; turn in
Insomnia	Awake half the night; can't get off (to sleep); sleeplessness; wakefulness; wide awake
Narcolepsy	Drop off without warning
Sleep	Catnap; doze/dozing off; drop off; forty winks; kip; lose myself; nap; siesta; shut eye; snooze
Sleep hygiene	Bed time or pre-sleep routine/rituals
Somnambulance[72]	Sleep walking
Somnolent	Dozy; drowsy; heavy-eyed; nodding off; sleepy
Weary	Dead beat; dog-tired; done in; ready to drop; whacked

71. hit the hay「寝る」かつて, hay「干し草」でベッドを作ったことから, hay に hit「体を当てる」で go to bed を意味する。同様に, hit the sack「床につく」は sack「綿の入った袋, マットレス」に hit「体を当てる」。
72. somnambulance「夢遊[症]」同様の表現に, somnambulism, neirodynia activa などもある。

Unit 10　　　　　　　　　　　　　　　　　　　　　　　　　睡眠

睡眠に関連する看護・医学用語あるいは標準英語，並びにそれと対応する口語的な用語と表現が Box. 8 にまとめられている。

注記：病歴と会話例文中における口語的な表現には，〔　〕内に説明を加えた。

BOX. 8

睡眠に関連した語

看護・医療用語 または標準的な用語	患者が使う口語的（日常的） または，俗語の（非常にくだけた）用語と表現
歯ぎしり	寝ている間に歯を擦り合わせる
ベッドに入る/ 就寝する	寝る・床につく，就寝する，お休みと言う，床につく
不眠〔症〕	夜中まで起きている, 眠れない, 不眠症, 覚醒状態, すっかり目が覚めている
ナルコレプシー	突然寝入る
睡眠	うたた寝, うたた寝する［している］, 居眠り, うたた寝, 眠り, 眠る, ぼんやりする, 昼寝, 眠ること, 居眠り
睡眠衛生	就寝［就寝前］の習慣［決まりごと］
夢遊〔症〕	夢遊〔病〕
傾眠〔傾眠の〕	眠そうな, うとうとして, 瞼が重い, 居眠りしている, 眠い
疲れ果てた	疲れ果てた, くたくたに疲れた, 疲れきっている, 疲れ果てて, 疲れた

Case history 14   Sleep deprivation: Mrs Bell

Mrs Bell moved into the care home[73] from sheltered housing[74] [housing with communal areas[75] and a warden] 5 days ago. She had enjoyed her time there, but after the fall and the fractured hip she felt that she needed more care. Although there was a button to press to get help, she was frightened of falling again and having to wait for help to come. Both her sons were concerned about her and going into the home seemed the most sensible thing to do. She hadn't expected to feel at home straight away, but she is missing her friends and is not sleeping well.

🔘 15

Nurse: Good morning Mrs Bell how are you settling in?
Mrs B.: Not too bad I suppose, but it feels a bit strange still.
Nurse: I thought it would be helpful for us to have a chat now that you have been here for a few days. You said that it feels strange.
Mrs B.: I'm not complaining and everyone is so kind, but I miss the ladies from the sheltered housing.
Nurse: Have any of them visited you yet?
Mrs B.: The warden came yesterday and it was nice to hear all the gossip. My special friends are away on their hols [holiday][76] until next week, so I expect they will be round then.
Nurse: That's good. What about your sons?
Mrs B.: John brought me in, and he came yesterday on his way home from work. Nigel works away during the week, but he will be in on Saturday.
Nurse: Have you got to know the other residents yet?
Mrs B.: I had tea [a light meal in the afternoon or evening] with Mrs

---

73.care home「(英国英語で, 高齢者・病人などが居住できる) 介護・保護施設」
74.sheltered housing「シェルタード・ハウジング」英国の, 高齢者向けの小規模の集合住宅。住み込みのスタッフがいるが, 基本的には重度の看護を必要としない人が居住する。
75.communal area「共同部分」
76.away on holiday「休暇を取って〔不在である〕」

症例14　　睡眠障害：ベル夫人

ベル夫人は，5日前にシェルタード・ハウジング［共同部分があり，管理人がいる住宅］から介護施設に引っ越した。彼女はそこでの生活を楽しんでいたが，転倒して股関節部を骨折してから，より多くの世話が必要だと感じるようになった。そこには助けを呼ぶためのボタンはあったが，彼女はもう一度転倒することや，助けてもらうまで待たなければならないことを怖がった。息子は2人とも彼女のことを心配し，介護施設に入居することが最も良い判断であると思っている。もともとすぐに施設に慣れるとは思ってはいなかったものの，やはり友達を懐かしみ，よく眠れないでいる。

看護師：　おはようございます，ベルさん。ここには慣れてきましたか？

B夫人：　そんなに悪くないと思います。でもまだ慣れない感じはしますね。

看護師：　ここに来て数日になるので，2人で少しおしゃべりするのはいいことだと思うんです。まだ慣れない感じがするとおっしゃいましたね。

B夫人：　不平を言っているわけではありませんし，みなさんとても親切です。でも，シェルタード・ハウジングの女友達がいなくて寂しくて。

看護師：　まだどなたも訪ねて来ませんか？

B夫人：　管理人さんは昨日来ました。いろいろなうわさ話が聞けて楽しかったです。特に仲の良いお友達は旅行［holsはholiday「休暇，休暇旅行」の略］で来週までいないので，そのころに来るのではないかと思います。

看護師：　それはいいですね。息子さんたちはいかがですか？

B夫人：　ジョンは私をここへ連れて来てくれて，昨日は仕事の帰りに寄ってくれました。ナイジェルは平日は遠くで働いているけれど，土曜日に来てくれるでしょう。

看護師：　ほかの入居者の方たちと知り合いになりましたか？

B夫人：　フォーブス夫人とお茶［午後や夕方の軽い食事］をいただきました。

		Forbes and she was very friendly.
	Nurse:	How are you sleeping?
20	Mrs B.:	Not very well, I'm awake half the night.
	Nurse:	Is that usual for you?
	Mrs B.:	Not really. I used to have the odd [in this context means 'infrequent' or 'unusual'] night when I would wake up, but most nights I would sleep right through until about half past
25		six [6.30 a.m.].
	Nurse:	Do you have trouble falling asleep [going to sleep] or do you wake up in the night?
	Mrs B.:	I'm really tired, but as soon as I put the light out[77] I'm wide awake again.
30	Nurse:	Do you get to sleep eventually?
	Mrs B.:	Yes, but then I wake up feeling whacked [weary] and groggy[78] [unwell]. I don't feel rested.
	Nurse:	Do you wake up earlier than usual?
	Mrs B.:	I did this morning. There was a lot of coming and going
35		[activity] because the lady in the next room was poorly [unwell].
	Nurse:	Yes, she had to go into hospital.
	Mrs B.:	And I'm so tired in the day I keep dozing off[79] [going to sleep] in the chair.
40	Nurse:	Did you usually have a short nap [sleep] during the day before you came to us?
	Mrs B.:	Well, if I'm honest, I did sometimes put my feet up [relax] after the lunchtime Archers [a long-running radio programme] and lose myself for a bit [have a short sleep].
45	Nurse:	What time have you been falling asleep in the chair?
	Mrs B.:	After supper [last meal of the day], so when I come to[80] [wake

77. put the light out「明かりを消す, 消灯する」
78. groggy「ぼんやりする, 足元がふらつく, 意識がもうろうとした」
79. doze off「うたた寝する, まどろむ」
80. come to「意識が戻る」

	彼女はとても親切でした。
看護師：	睡眠はいかがですか？
B夫人：	あまり良くありません。夜中まで目が覚めています。
看護師：	いつものことですか？
B夫人：	いいえ違います。目が覚めてしまう，おかしな［ここでの文脈では「めったにない」または「珍しい」という意味］夜もありましたが，ほとんどは6時半［午前6時30分］までぐっすり眠れていました。
看護師：	なかなか眠りにつけない［寝付けない］のですか。それとも夜中に目が覚めるのですか？
B夫人：	とても疲れているのに，明かりを消すとまたすぐにすっかり目が覚めてしまいます。
看護師：	最後には眠れますか？
B夫人：	はい，でも起きたときにはとても疲れていて［疲労して］ぼんやりします［具合が悪いです］。休めた気がしません。
看護師：	普通より早く起きますか？
B夫人：	今朝はそうでした。隣の女性の調子が悪く［具合が悪く］，行き来が激しかった［活発だった］のです。
看護師：	ええ，彼女は入院しなければなりませんでした。
B夫人：	そして日中にあまりに疲れるので，ひじ掛椅子でうとうとして［寝て］ばかりいます。
看護師：	ここに来る前，いつも日中に昼寝をして［ひと眠りして］いましたか？
B夫人：	ええ，正直に言うと，お昼の『アーチャー』［長年続いているラジオ番組］の後に足を伸ばして［リラックス］して少しぼんやりすることがありました［休むことがありました］。
看護師：	椅子でうたた寝するのは何時ごろですか？
B夫人：	夕食［1日の最後の食事］の後です。それで，意識が戻った［目覚めた］

	up] it's time to start thinking about going to bed. That's a bit late for a nap I know.
Nurse:	Do you have a bedtime routine — things that help you get to sleep?
Mrs B.:	I used to have a bath last thing [just before going to bed] and take a milky drink to bed. Then read until I felt drowsy[81] [somnolent].
Nurse:	What sort of time [approximate timing] would you usually have the bath?
Mrs B.:	After the news at ten [10 p.m.] and be in bed by 11 [11 p.m.]. I'm not sure if it's all right to have a bath that late here. I expect the girls [night staff] are too busy to help with baths.
Nurse:	I will have a word [discuss it] with the nurse in charge tonight about making sure you can have a bath if you want, and get a milky drink. It is so important to get a good night's sleep.
Mrs B.:	You can say that again [emphasises the importance of the nurse's last statement]. I would be very grateful if they could help me with a bath.
Nurse:	Is there anything else that can be done to help you sleep properly?
Mrs B.:	It is quite warm in my room. I'm not used to having the radiator so hot in the bedroom.
Nurse:	We can turn the thermostat down, so it just takes the chill off the room [make sure that the room is not cold].
Mrs B.:	They tried last night, but it was too stiff to turn.
Nurse:	I'll get on to [contact] the maintenance staff right away [at once].
Mrs B.:	It was so hot I pushed the duvet off me. I haven't done that

---

81.drowsy「眠い、うとうとして」

ときには，もう寝ることを考える時間になっています。昼寝には少し遅い時間だということはわかってはいるのですが。

看護師： 眠りやすくなるような，寝る前の習慣は何かありますか？

B夫人： 以前は最後に［ベッドに入る直前］にお風呂に入って，ベッドに乳飲料を持って行きました。それから，うとうとする［眠気を誘われる］まで本を読んだものです。

看護師： どんな時間に［何時頃］にいつも入浴したいですか。

B夫人： 10時［午後10時］のニュースの後です。そして11時［午後11時］までにベッドに入るようにしたいです。ここではそんなに遅く入浴してもよいのかわかりませんけど。おじょうさんたち［夜勤のスタッフ］は忙しくて入浴の介助はできないでしょうね。

看護師： 今夜の担当の看護師と話し［話し合い］ます。ご希望でしたら入浴して，乳飲料を飲めるようにしておきます。夜にきちんと睡眠を取るのはとても大切です。

B夫人： まったくそのとおりです［看護師の最後の言葉の重要性を強調している］。もし入浴を手伝っていただけるならとてもうれしいです。

看護師： よく眠れるようにするため，ほかにできることはありますか？

B夫人： 部屋がとても暖かいです。こんなに寝室を暖房で暖かくするのには慣れていません。

看護師： 少し温める程度に［部屋が寒くはないように］温度自動調節器〔の設定温度〕を下げましょう。

B夫人： 昨晩試してもらいました。でも，硬すぎて回せなかったのです。

看護師： 設備の担当者にすぐに［ただちに］話［連絡］をします。

		since the change[82] [climacteric[83]/menopause[84]] when I used to have night sweats.
	Nurse:	What about when you get up in the morning, will you be warm enough?
80	Mrs B.:	Oh yes, my boys [her sons] treated me to [paid for] some new clothes to come in here and that included a fleecy dressing gown. Look it's on the chair. Do you think it's too bright?
	Nurse:	I like that dark pink. It's such a warm colour.
85	Mrs B.:	Yes, I like it. I did wonder about pink at my age, but then I thought 'Why not?'.
	Nurse:	Is there anything else that stops you sleeping?
	Mrs B.:	I still need to get used to [become accustomed to] the light coming in from the corridor.
90	Nurse:	Were you used to sleeping in complete darkness?
	Mrs B.:	Yes, the sheltered housing is on the edge of the village, right out in the sticks [rural location, in the countryside].
	Nurse:	We need to keep the light on in the corridor, so that everyone can move about[34] safely.
95	Mrs B.:	Yes, I know. I don't suppose it will bother [trouble] me for long.

---

82. the change「閉経期」
83. climacteric「閉経期〔の〕」
84. menopause「更年期, 月経閉止, 閉経」
(**34. move about**「あちこち動き回る」)

B夫人：	とても暑くて掛け布団をはいでしまいました。そんなことをするのは更年期［更年期，閉経期］のとき寝汗をかいていたとき以来です。
看護師：	朝起きたときはいかがですか。十分に暖かいですか？
B夫人：	大丈夫です。うちの子たち［彼女の息子たち］がここに来るときに新しい服をプレゼントして［買って］くれて，その中にふわふわした部屋着もありました。椅子の上にあるのを見て。〔色が〕明るすぎます？
看護師：	ダークピンクはいいですね。とても温かみのある色です。
B夫人：	ええ，私も好きなんです。私の年でピンクなんてどうかと思いましたが，その後で，「別にいいじゃない」って思って。
看護師：	ほかに睡眠の邪魔になることはありますか？
B夫人：	廊下から入ってくる明かりも慣れ［習慣とし］なければなりません。
看護師：	これまでは真っ暗な中で寝ていましたか？
B夫人：	はい，シェルタード・ハウジングは辺鄙な所［田舎，地方］の村の外れでしたから。
看護師：	みんなが安全にあちこち動けるように，廊下はずっと明るくしておかなければならないんです。
B夫人：	ええ，わかっています。長くは気［問題］にならないでしょう。

Unit 11 WORKING AND PLAYING

Some nursing/medical or Standard English words and corresponding colloquial words and expressions associated with working and playing are given in Box. 9.

Note: Colloquial expressions used in the case histories and example conversations are explained in brackets [...].

BOX. 9

Words associated with working and playing

Nursing/medical or Standard English words	Colloquial (everyday) or slang (very informal) words and expressions used by patients
Dismissed	Fired; given my cards; given the boot; given my notice; given the push; got the sack; laid off; let go; marching orders; sacked; sent packing
Employed	Hired; in a job; in work; paid work; working
Employee	Bread-winner; wage-earner; worker
Employer	Boss; gaffer; governor
Leisure/leisure activities	Amusement; breathing space; free time; fun; hobby; pastime; play; pleasure; recreation; R&R; spare time; time off
Occupation; profession	Business; career; calling (outdated); craft; job; line of work; livelihood; position; trade; walk of life; work
Relaxation	Chill out; laze about; let one's hair down; loosen up; put one's feet up; take it easy; unwind
Retired	Given up work; pensioner; pensioned off; put out to grass
Self-employed	Freelance; my own boss; work for myself
Unemployed	Jobless; looking for a job/work; not working; on the dole/social; out of work

Unit 11　　　　　　　　　　　　　　　　　　　　　仕事と遊び

仕事と遊びに関連する看護・医学用語あるいは標準英語，並びにそれと対応する口語的な用語と表現が Box. 9 にまとめられている。

注記：病歴と会話例文中における口語的な表現には，〔　〕内に説明を加えた。

BOX. 9
仕事と遊びに関連する用語

看護／医学用語，または標準英語の用語	患者が使う, 口語的（日常的な）または, 俗語の（非常にくだけた）用語と表現
解雇された	首になった；雇用書類〔雇い主が預かっていて退職時に返す〕を渡された；〔雇用主などに〕不要だと言われた；〔解雇の〕通告を与えられた；首にされた；首になった；一時解雇された；解雇された；解雇通告；首になった；首を切られて
雇われている	雇われた；仕事に就いて；就職して；賃金労働；働いている
従業員	稼ぎ手〔大黒柱〕；賃金労働者；労働者
雇用主	社長；親方；親分
余暇／余暇活動	娯楽；息をつく時間；自由な時間；楽しみ；趣味；気晴らし；遊び；楽しみ；娯楽；保養休暇〔Rest & Recreation〕；空き時間；休み
職／職業	仕事；〔生涯の〕職業；天職（古い言い回し）；〔特殊技術を要する〕仕事；仕事；職種；生計；職；〔特別な技術を要する〕職業；職業〔階層〕；仕事
気晴らし	のんびり過ごす；ゆったり過ごす；くつろぐ；リラックスする；〔両足を何かに乗せて〕くつろぐ；のんびりする；緊張が解ける
退職して	仕事を辞めて；年金生活［受給］者；年金を与えられて退職して；引退して
自営の	フリーで働く人；独立して働いている；自営業をしている
失業している	仕事の無い；仕事／仕事を探している；働いていない；失業手当／生活保護を受けて；失業している

Case history 15   After myocardial infarction: Mr Khan

Mr Khan is about to[85] be discharged home after having a myocardial infarction a week ago. He normally helps to run the family business and needs to drive all over the UK to see customers. He is anxious about how a recent myocardial infarction will affect his driving, the business and his leisure activities.

🔊 16

Mr K.:	Nurse Brown, have you got a minute [the time] to talk?
Nurse:	I need to give a painkiller to another patient. I'll be back in 5 minutes.
Mr K.:	OK.
Nurse:	Right, Mr Khan I'm back. What would you like to talk about?
Mr K.:	I'm really worried about how I'll manage to run[86] my part of the business after the heart attack [myocardial infarction].
Nurse:	Did you speak to the cardiac nurse specialist?
Mr K.:	Yes, on Tuesday. She explained everything and I asked lots of questions. It all seemed quite straightforward [easy, simple], but now that I'm dressed and ready to go home I'm not so sure.
Nurse:	Did she leave the printed information?
Mr K.:	Yes.
Nurse:	What bits are worrying you?
Mr K.:	Well, mainly the driving and getting back to work. I drive about 20,000 miles a year on business. There is something in the leaflet about driving, but I'm worried that Swansea [the location of the Driver and Vehicle Licensing Agency (DVLA); the word 'Swansea' may be used to describe it in conversation] will take my licence away.

85. is about to ...「まさに〜するところで」
86. run ...「〜を行う,切り盛りする」

症例15　心筋梗塞のその後：カーン氏

カーン氏は1週間前に心筋梗塞になり，これから退院するところである。彼は通常であれば家業の手伝いをしており，顧客と会うために英国中を車で行く必要がある。彼が心配しているのは，この心筋梗塞で運転・仕事・余暇活動にどのような影響が出るかということである。

K氏：　　ブラウン看護師，ちょっとの間[時間]話せますか？

看護師：　ほかの患者さんに痛み止めをあげないといけないんです。5分で戻ります。

K氏：　　わかりました。

看護師：　はい，カーンさん，戻りました。お話ししたいことというのは何でしょう？

K氏：　　心臓発作[心筋梗塞]の後で，どうやって仕事の私の分担分をやっていくかということがとても心配です。

看護師：　心臓専門の看護師に話しましたか？

K氏：　　はい，火曜日に。彼女はいろいろ説明してくれて，私もたくさん質問しました。みんなとてもわかりやすい[簡単，やさしい]と思ったんですが，いざ服を着て家に帰るとなると，なんだか自信がなくて。

看護師：　彼女は資料をくれましたか？

K氏：　　はい。

看護師：　どんなところが心配ですか？

K氏：　　そうですね，主に運転と，仕事に戻る点です。仕事で1年間に2万マイル運転します。その案内には運転について書いてありますが，スウォンジー[運転者・車両免許局（DVLA）のある地名；Swansea「スウォンジー」という単語はそれを表現するのに慣習的に使われることがある]に，免許を取り上げられるのではないかと心配しています。

	Nurse:	Is yours an ordinary licence?
	Mr K.:	I should think so.
25	Nurse:	You don't drive a bus or a lorry do you?
	Mr K.:	No, just the car and sometimes the minibus for the Community Centre.
	Nurse:	You will need to stop driving for at least 4 weeks and you don't have to notify DVLA. You have an appointment to see Dr Bradley [the cardiologist] next month. He will advise you about when you can start driving again.
30		
	Mr K.:	I hope it's not much longer than 4 weeks. My dad [father] and brother can visit the customers for a few weeks, but not for ever.
35	Nurse:	So far your recovery has gone well. There's no reason to think you won't be fit [well enough] to drive in a month. It might be a good idea to tell your insurance company about the heart attack.
	Mr K.:	Yes, that's sensible. I don't want to drive without insurance. That means a fine and six points on your licence[87].
40		
	Nurse:	You mentioned getting back to work.
	Mr K.:	We run a small family business, so one person off sick puts a real strain on everyone else.
	Nurse:	Yes, I can see that. Do you do most of the customer visiting?
45	Mr K.:	Yes, my dad doesn't really like driving long distances and my brother is better at the day-to-day business.
	Nurse:	Again Dr Bradley will advise you about going back to work, but most people gradually increase their activity and are back at work in 4-6 weeks. It would be longer if you had a job with a lot of physical activity.
50		
	Mr K.:	No, if I'm in the office it's mainly computer work and telephoning customers. My job isn't very active, but I'm

---

87.six points on your licence「免許に 6 ポイント加算」英国では違反の点数が 1 から 12 まであり、違反をすると違反の種類を表すコードと、違反の点数が免許に書かれる。

看護師： 免許は普通免許ですか？

K氏： そう思いますが。

看護師： バスや大型トラックは運転しないんでしょう？

K氏： はい，ただ〔普通の〕車と，たまにコミュニティ・センターのためにミニバスを運転するだけです。

看護師： 少なくとも4週間は運転できませんが，DVLAに知らせる必要はありません。ブラッドリー先生〔心臓専門医〕に来月予約がありますね。いつ運転できるようになるかアドバイスがもらえますよ。

K氏： 4週間より延びなければいいんですが。何週間かは父さん〔父〕と兄弟がお客さんのところに行けますが，ずっとではありませんから。

看護師： 今のところ回復は順調です。1か月後に運転できるくらいに〔運転するのに十分良く〕なっていると考えるのが自然ですよ。加入している保険会社には心臓発作のことを伝えておいたほうがいいですね。

K氏： そうですね，賢明です。保険なしで運転したくありませんから。罰金と，免許に6ポイント加算になりますからね。

看護師： 仕事に戻ることについて触れましたね。

K氏： 小さな家族経営なので，1人が病気でいなくなるとほかのみんなにすごく負担がかかってしまうんです。

看護師： そうですね，わかります。あなたが顧客訪問をほとんどやっているんですか？

K氏： そうです，父さんは長距離の運転があまり好きではないし，兄弟は日常業務のほうが得意なんです。

看護師： この場合も，ブラッドリー先生が仕事復帰についてアドバイスしてくれるでしょうけど，たいていの人は徐々に活動を増やしていって，4週間から6週間で仕事に戻ります。肉体労働が多い仕事ならもっと長くなるでしょうけど。

K氏： いいえ，事務所にいるときはコンピュータ仕事やお客さんへの電話業務が中心です。仕事はそれほど活動的ではありませんが，スポーツを

		keen on[88] sport.
	Nurse:	What sport do you do?
55	Mr K.:	I play some cricket and coach some lads [boys, youngsters] in a local football team.
	Nurse:	How active is the coaching?
	Mr K.:	Well I work-out [train] with the boys. I'm keen to keep[89] on [continue] with both the cricket and the coaching.
60	Nurse:	The staff running [organising] the formal sessions of the cardiac rehabilitation programme will be able to give you information about safe levels of exercise and playing sport. When do you start?
	Mr K.:	The specialist nurse said that she will give me a ring [telephone] next week to see how we're getting on [coping] at home and by then she will know the dates for the exercise sessions.
65		
	Nurse:	Don't forget the cardiac nurses have a telephone helpline if you have any worries once you get home, and you can also use their e-mail.
70		
	Mr K.:	Yes, it's very reassuring to know that there is some back-up [support].
	Nurse:	Have you any questions about your drugs and the dietary changes, or anything else?
75	Mr K.:	No, that's all the worries for now. I just needed to get those things straight [sorted] in my mind.

---

88. be keen on ...「〜に熱心で」
89. be keen to do ...「熱心に〜をしたがる」

熱心にしています。
看護師： どういうスポーツをするんですか？
K氏： クリケットと，地元のサッカーチームで若いやつら［少年，若者］のコーチをしています。
看護師： コーチというのはどれくらい活動的なんですか？
K氏： そうですね，彼らと一緒に運動［練習］します。クリケットとコーチの両方はぜひ続けたい［持続したい］と思っています。
看護師： 心臓リハビリプログラムの正式な研修会を運営している［開催している］スタッフが，安全なレベルの運動とスポーツについて情報をくれますよ。いつ始めますか？
K氏： 専門看護師が，私が自宅でどんな風にやっているか［対処しているか］確認するため，来週電話［電話］をくれるそうです。そのときまでには，運動研修会の日にちも決まるだろうと言っていました。
看護師： 家に帰って何か心配になったら，心臓専門看護師の電話ヘルプラインを忘れないで。それに，メールでも相談できます。
K氏： はい，支援［サポート］があると思うととても安心します。
看護師： 薬や，食事の変更，その他のことで何か質問はありますか？
K氏： いいえ，今のところお話ししたことが心配ごとのすべてです。ただこういうことを頭の中で整理［きちんと］しないといけなかったんです。

Case history 16   Diabetic retinopathy: Mrs Hamilton

Mrs Hamilton has had diabetes for many years and her vision is deteriorating[90] due to[91] diabetic retinopathy. She and her husband are both retired and enjoy walking and gardening.

17

Nurse: Hello Mrs Hamilton. It doesn't seem like a year since we last saw you.

Mrs H.: Yes, time for the annual eye check again.

Nurse: Not everyone is so reliable about attending as you.

5 Mrs H.: I'd be daft [foolish, unwise] not to. Finding problems early is so important. My Sight is already bad, I don't want it to get any worse.

Nurse: I will be putting the eye drops in to dilate your pupil, so we can examine the back of your eye [retina]. How has your sight been since last year's check?

Mrs H.: I'm finding it more difficult to read small print and I've got patchy [uneven] blurring of vision. It does make life difficult.

Nurse: How does it affect you on a day-to-day basis?

Mrs H.: Now Jim [her husband] and I have given up working [retired] we have time to do our garden. I have always had green fingers [keen gardener] and we like walking in the countryside, but it's not much fun with my poor vision. I have to rely on Jim to read the labels on weed killer for the garden and the plant labels at the garden centre. He doesn't mind, but I mind very much. I feel so helpless and frustrated about losing my independence.

Nurse: Yes, it must be frustrating.

Mrs H.: I'm really cheesed off [fed up]. It's reading books as well. I like to relax with a book after supper [last meal of the day]

90. deteriorate「低下する, 悪化する」
91. due to ...「〜のために」

★   130

症例 16　　糖尿病性網膜症：ハミルトン夫人

ハミルトン夫人は何年も糖尿病を患っていて，糖尿病性網膜症のために視力が低下している。彼女と夫は2人とも退職していて，散歩とガーデニングを楽しんでいる。

看護師：　こんにちは，ハミルトンさん。最後にお会いしてから1年が経ったなんて思えませんね。

H夫人：　ええ，また毎年恒例の眼の検査の時期ですよ。

看護師：　こんなに確実に検査を受けてくれる人はそういませんよ。

H夫人：　検査を受けないなんてばかばかしい［ばかげた，賢明ではない］ことですよ。問題の早期発見はとても重要です。すでに視力が悪いので，これ以上ひどくしたくありません。

看護師：　瞳孔を広げるために眼薬をさしますね。眼の後ろ［網膜］が調べられますから。去年の検査以降，視力はいかがですか？

H夫人：　小さな文字がより見づらくなっています。それから，視界がまだらに［一様ではなく］ぼやけます。そのせいで本当に困っています。

看護師：　日常的にはどう影響していますか？

H夫人：　今はジム［彼女の夫］と私は仕事をしていない［退職している］ので，ガーデニングをする時間があるんです。私はずっと園芸が得意［ガーデニングに熱心な人］で，2人とも田舎を散歩するのが好きなんですが，視力が良くないとそれほど楽しめません。庭で使う除草剤のラベルを読んだり，園芸用品店で植物のラベルを読んだりするのをジムに頼らないとならないんです。彼は気にしてませんが，私にはとても気になります。自立できなくなっていくのが心細くて，いらいらするんです。

看護師：　わかります，ストレスでしょう。

H夫人：　本当にうんざり［いやになるん］です。本を読むのも同じです。夕食［1

25		while Jim has a pint[92] [in this context it means beer] at our local [nearest public house]. But now I can only see if the print is very large and every light in the room is on. It's not very relaxing.
	Nurse:	No, it doesn't sound very relaxing. Have you got any low vision aids?
30	Mrs H.:	I've got my glasses [spectacles] and a magnifier and I make sure that the lighting is right for what I'm doing.
	Nurse:	How is your diabetic control?
	Mrs H.:	OK. I'm doing quite well with the sugar control and the insulin injections are no problem now I use a preloaded insulin pen [device for injecting insulin].
35		
	Nurse:	I'm sure you know how important this is to help stop the retinopathy from getting worse.
	Mrs H.:	Oh yes, the diabetic nurse specialists are always harping on about [emphasising] the importance of managing the diabetes properly.
40		
	Nurse:	We all nag [keep on at] you, don't we?
	Mrs H.:	I don't mind. But just think, if I hadn't gone after [applied for] the area manager post [job] and had to have a medical [routine health check] it might have been ages [long time] before they found the diabetes and I started the insulin and a proper diet.
45		

---

92. a pint「〔生ビールの〕1 杯」英国では生ビールをパイントのグラスで頼む。2 分の 1 の量のグラスで飲むハーフ・パイントという頼み方もある。

日の最後の食事]の後，ジムが近所［1番近いパブ］で1杯飲む［ここではビールを意味する］間，私は本を読んでリラックスするのが好きなんです。でも，今は文字がとても大きくないといけないし，部屋の明かりもすべてつけなければ見えないんです。あんまりリラックスできません。

看護師： そうですね，そんなにリラックスできるとは思えないですね。低視力用の補助器具は何かお持ちですか？

H夫人： 眼鏡［眼鏡］と拡大鏡を持っています。それから，必ず自分がすることに合わせてちょうどよい明るさに調整するようにしています。

看護師： 糖尿病の管理はどんな感じですか？

H夫人： 大丈夫です。糖のコントロールはけっこううまくいっているし，インシュリンがあらかじめ入っているペン型の注射器［インシュリンを注射する道具］を使っているので，インシュリンの注射も今では問題ありません。

看護師： このことが網膜症の悪化を防ぐのにどんなに重要かよくご存知だと思います。

H夫人： ええ，もちろんです。糖尿病の専門看護師は，糖尿病の適切な管理の重要さをいつでもくどくどと言います［強調しています］。

看護師： 私たちはみんなうるさく言いますでしょう？

H夫人： いいんですよ。でも，考えてもみて，もし私がエリア・マネジャーの職［仕事］をしようとしないで［応募しないで］健康診断［定期健康診断］も受けなくてすんでいたら，糖尿病が見つかってインシュリンとちゃんとした食事を始めるまでに何年も［長い時間］かかったかもしれませんよ。

Unit 12 SEXUALITY

Some nursing/medical or Standard English words and corresponding colloquial words and expressions associated with sexuality are given in Box. 10.

Note: Colloquial expressions used in the case histories and example conversations are explained in brackets [...].

BOX. 10

Words associated with sexuality

Nursing/medical or Standard English words	Colloquial (everyday) or slang (very informal) words and expressions used by patients
Cervix	Neck of womb
Dysmenorrhoea	Painful periods
Erectile dysfunction	Impotent
Genitalia	Bits; down below; down there, naughty bits; private parts; privates
Menorrhagia	Flooding; heavy periods
Menstruation	Being unwell; having the curse. period(s)
Sexual intercourse	Go to bed with; intimacy; lovemaking; make love; sex; sexual relations; sleep with; to do/have it
Uterus	Womb

Case history 17   Erectile dysfunction: Mr Johns

Mr Johns has been a widower [a man whose wife has died and has not remarried] for many years. He is generally fit [in good health], apart from hypertension which is treated with enalapril maleate.

Unit 12　　　　　　　　　　　　　　　　　　　　　　　　　性

性に関連する看護・医学用語あるいは標準英語，並びにそれと対応する口語的な用語と表現が Box. 10 にまとめられている。

注記：病歴と会話例文中における口語的な表現には，［　］内に説明を加えた。

BOX. 10

性に関連する用語

看護／医学用語， 標準的英語の用語	患者が使う口語的（日常的） または，俗語の（非常にくだけた）単語と表現
子宮頚部	子宮の頚部
月経困難	苦痛を伴う月経
勃起障害	勃起しない
性器	性器；下の方；下の方，エッチな部分；あの部分；あそこ
月経過多〔症〕	大量出血する；重い月経
月経	生理中である；生理である，生理
性交	〜とベッドに行く；性的な関係；セックスすること；セックス；性交；肉体関係；〜と寝る；〔セックスを〕やる／する
子宮	子宮

症例 17　　勃起障害：ジョンズ氏

ジョンズ氏は何年も男やもめ［妻に先立たれて再婚していない］である。彼は，マレイン酸エナラプリルで治療中の高血圧を除いては，全般的に元気［健康］である。

Mr J.:	I've been under the doctor [in the doctor's care, being treated] for my blood pressure. She said to make an appointment for you to check me over and do the blood pressure.
Nurse:	What has the doctor prescribed?
Mr J.:	Innovace [proprietary name for enalapril maleate].
Nurse:	How have you been?
Mr J.:	Not bad [In English, when you have two negatives, known as a 'double negative,' it creates a middle way, meaning not a positive ('very good'), but not a negative ('very bad') either].
Nurse:	What, not feeling really well?
Mr J.:	A bit seedy [unwell], but nothing specific.
Nurse:	Is there anything worrying you?
Mr J.:	I've met a nice lady, we really hit it off [get on well]. She likes all the same things as me, music, food and everything.
Nurse:	Had you been on your own for long?
Mr J.:	A long time. Jenny [his wife] died of cancer 10 years ago. I didn't want anyone else at first, but when the kids [children] married and moved away I felt a bit lonely and that.
Nurse:	Yes.
Mr J.:	I met someone at work, but that soon fizzled out [came to nothing].
Nurse:	Some men can have difficulty with erections when taking the medicine you are on. Have you had any trouble?
Mr J.:	It's difficult to talk about it, but I was impotent [had erectile dysfunction] and couldn't do it [have sexual intercourse]. I told myself it was just nerves being with someone new and tiredness.
Nurse:	Yes, it's difficult to talk about intimate things.

J氏：	血圧で医者にかかっています［医者の世話になっている，治療している］。彼女に，検査と血圧の測定をあなたに予約するよう言われました。
看護師：	医師は何を処方していますか？
J氏：	イノベース［マイレン酸エナラプリルの商標名］です。
看護師：	具合はどうですか？
J氏：	悪くはないです［英語では，「二重否定」として知られているが，2つの否定語を使うと，中間の意味となる。つまり，肯定的（「とてもよい」）ではないが，否定的（「とても悪い」）でもない］。
看護師：	えっ，あんまりよくないんですか？
J氏：	ちょっと調子が悪い［具合が悪い］けど，どこがというわけではありません。
看護師：	何か心配ごとでもおありですか？
J氏：	素敵な女性と出会いました。本当に馬が合うんです［気が合うんです］。私が好きなことはみんな彼女も好きなんです，音楽，食事，何もかも。
看護師：	長い間お1人でしたか？
J氏：	長い間ね。10年前にジェニー［彼の妻］ががんで他界しました。最初はほかのだれとも会いたいとは思わなかったんです。でも，子供たち［子供たち］が結婚して出て行ったとき，ちょっと寂しいというか，そんな風なことを感じました。
看護師：	なるほど。
J氏：	職場で出会った人もいましたが，すぐに立ち消えになりました［実を結びませんでした］。
看護師：	あなたが処方されている薬を服用する男性の中には，勃起に障害が出る人もいます。何かトラブルはありますか？
J氏：	言いづらいんですけど，性的に不能［勃起障害］で，あれができませんでした［性交渉が持てませんでした］。新しい人と一緒にいて神経質になっているだけだ，疲れのせいだ，と自分に言い聞かせました。
看護師：	そうですね，個人的な事柄は話しづらいですよね。

	Mr J.:	I'm worried about my new relationship. I don't want anything to go wrong like last time.
	Nurse:	We're lucky in this area to have a nurse who specialises in the management of erectile dysfunction, that's the medical term for problems with erections. Would you like me to arrange an assessment appointment with him?
	Mr J.:	Yes please, I need to talk to someone. When the doctor gave me the script [short for prescription] she said one of the side-effects was trouble with erections, but how could I ask her any questions? It was so embarrassing.

Case history 18   Dysmenorrhoea: Mrs Hall

Problems with menstruation have been part of Mrs Hall's life for as long as she can remember. First it was dysmenorrhoea as a teenager and into her 20s, and now 20 years later she has menorrhagia and the dysmenorrhoea is back. She has seen the consultant and the plan is for her to come in as a day case for a hysteroscopy and endometrial biopsy.

19

Nurse:	Hello again Mrs Hall. I've come to answer any questions you might have about having the examination as a day case.
Mrs H.:	You and the consultant explained that he would look inside the womb [uterus] with a special instrument and then do a scrape [dilatation and curettage] to get a sample for testing, so I'm fairly clear about what will happen.
Nurse:	Have you any questions about the possible complications of the procedure?
Mrs H.:	No, I'm fully aware that there is a risk of the womb being perforated.

J氏:	新しい恋愛関係が心配です。この前のように失敗したくはないんです。
看護師:	この分野において私たちはラッキーですよ。勃起障害，これは勃起の問題を表す医療用語ですが，それを専門とする看護師がいますから。彼に意見を聞く予約をしましょうか？
J氏:	ええ，お願いします。だれかに相談する必要があります。医者がスクリプト［scrip は prescription「処方箋」の略］をくれたとき，副作用の1つに勃起のトラブルがあると聞きましたが，彼女〔医者〕に質問なんてできませんでしたよ。とても恥ずかしくて。

症例18　月経困難：ホール夫人

ホール夫人が覚えている限り，月経の問題はずっと彼女の人生の一部だった。まず，10代から20代の頃は月経困難で，20年後の今は月経過多症となり，月経困難が再発した。彼女は専門医にかかっており，計画では，子宮内視鏡と子宮内膜の生検検査を日帰り処置として実施することになっている。

看護師:	ホールさん，こんにちは。今度は，日帰り検査を受けることで何か質問がおありでしたら，お答えしようと思って来ました。
H夫人:	あなたと専門医さんは，子宮［子宮］の内部を特別な機器で見て，それから検査のための検体をこすり取る［拡張と掻爬処置を行う］と説明してくれましたね。だから，どういうことになるのかだいたいわかっています。
看護師:	手術で起こるかもしれない合併症について質問はありますか？
H夫人:	いいえ，子宮に穴が開く危険性については十分承知しています。

	Nurse:	You signed your consent form and consented to a general anaesthetic.
	Mrs H.:	I didn't fancy [like the idea of] having it done in outpatients,
15		I'd rather be put to sleep [anaesthetised] first.
	Nurse:	It will only be a short anaesthetic. You should be able to go home later that afternoon/evening. Will your partner be collecting you?
	Mrs H.:	Yes, he'll come straight from work. His shift finishes at 3
20		o'clock, so it will be about 4 [4.00 p.m.]. Is that OK?
	Nurse:	No problem, but he should ring [telephone] first just to see if you are recovered enough to go home. You might still be a bit sleepy.
	Mrs H.:	Mr Bainbridge[93] said you could give me a date for the
25		examination.
	Nurse:	Yes, I'll get the dates up on the computer, but first I need to check a few things with you.
	Mrs H.:	OK.
	Nurse:	We do the examinations on a Wednesday morning. Are
30		there any dates that we need to avoid?
	Mrs H.:	No, we're not going away [in this context means away on holiday[76]] until the problems with my periods [menstruation] have been sorted out.
	Nurse:	We will need to avoid dates when you have your period, as
35		it makes it difficult to get a good view of the inside of the womb. Are your periods regular?
	Mrs H.:	Fairly. It usually comes every 30 days or so[94]. The real problem is that it lasts much longer.
	Nurse:	How long?

---

93. Mr. Bainbridge「ベインブリッジ先生」英国では外科医〔婦人科医も含む〕の敬称は Miss, Ms, Mrs, Mr で, Dr〔doctor「ドクター」〕ではない。かつて大学から与えられる外科専攻の学位が Doctor を名乗るものではなかったことから, 現在まで続いている。
94. or so「〜ばかり, ほど」数量・期間の表現に続けて用いる。
(**76. away on holiday**「休暇を取って〔不在である〕」)

看護師：	同意書への署名と，全身麻酔への同意はお済みですね。
H夫人：	外来では受けたくありませんでした〔〔受けること〕に反対でした〕。〔日帰りなら〕むしろ，最初に眠らせて〔全身麻酔をかけて〕くれるほうがありがたいです。
看護師：	ほんの短い麻酔です。その日の午後遅く／夕方，家に帰れるはずです。パートナーの方が迎えにいらっしゃいますか？
H夫人：	はい，職場から直接来ます。勤務シフトが3時に終わるので，4時〔午後4時〕くらいになります。それで大丈夫ですか？
看護師：	問題ありませんが，彼はまず電話して〔電話して〕あなたが家に帰れるくらいに回復しているか確認する必要があります。そのときまだちょっと眠いかもしれませんよ。
H夫人：	ベインブリッジ先生は検査の日程はあなたに教えてもらえると言っていました。
看護師：	はい，日程をコンピュータに出します。でも最初にいくつか確認しなければなりません。
H夫人：	いいですよ。
看護師：	ここでは水曜日の午前中に検査処置を行うことになっています。避ける必要がある日はありますか？
H夫人：	いいえ，私たちは生理〔月経〕の問題が解決するまでは出かけません〔この文脈では，休暇に出かけるという意味〕。
看護師：	子宮内部が良く見られなくなりますから，生理の間の日程は外さなければなりません。生理は規則的ですか？
H夫人：	かなり。30日毎かそれくらいで来ます。本当に問題なのは，とても長く続くことです。
看護師：	どのくらいですか？

40	Mrs H.:	The last 3 months have been dreadful, with the heavy bleeding going on for 7 or 8 days.
	Nurse:	Does that make things difficult for you?
	Mrs H.:	Yes, very difficult, because I keep flooding [excessive bleeding from the uterus]. Sometimes the blood comes through the pad and my clothes, so I'm scared [frightened] to go out. Plus I'm forever washing clothes and the bedding.
	Nurse:	It sounds as if your daily activities are seriously affected.
	Mrs H.:	Yes, they are. I can't plan to do anything for a whole week every month.
50	Nurse:	Do you have any spotting [intermenstrual bleeding], such as after having sexual intercourse?
	Mrs H.:	No, only the heavy bleeding [menorrhagia] and flooding during my period. But it's affecting our sex life; either I'm bleeding or too tired.
55	Nurse:	The blood test we took will show if you are anaemic. Heavy periods often cause anaemia and that would make you tired.
	Mrs H.:	I really want the bleeding sorted. It's really dragging me down [making me ill, emotionally and physically].
60	Nurse:	The examination will help to find a physical cause, but as you know Mr Bainbridge thinks that you may have dysfunctional uterine bleeding and he might not find a physical cause.
	Mrs H.:	I'm in agony [in extreme pain] with period pains [dysmenorrhoea] as well. I used to have pain with my periods when I was young, but this pain is much worse.
	Nurse:	What do you take for it?
	Mrs H.:	Just paracetamol, but they don't do much good [not very effective]. I know I said that I want it sorted, but I'm worried in case he says I need a hysterectomy.

H夫人：	ここ3か月はひどいものです。大量の出血が7日や8日も続きます。
看護師：	そのことでお困りですか？
H夫人：	ええ，とても困っています。ずっと大量に出血［子宮から過度に出血すること］し続けているからです。血が生理用ナプキンや服から滲み出ることがあって，外出するのが怖い［恐ろしい］です。その上，服と寝具類を延々と洗い続けてます。
看護師：	日常生活に深刻な影響が出ているようですね。
H夫人：	はい，そうなんです。毎月，まるまる1週間は何の予定も立てられません。
看護師：	生理の時期以外に血が混じること［中間期出血］はありますか，例えば，性行為の後のようなときに？
H夫人：	いいえ，生理のときに長い間出血すること［月経過多］と出血の量がとても多いことだけです。でも，セックスライフにも悪影響が出ています。出血しているか，疲れすぎているかのどちらかですから。
看護師：	以前行った血液検査で，貧血かどうか判明します。重い生理が貧血を起こすことはよくありますし，貧血だと疲れますから。
H夫人：	心から出血〔の問題〕を解決したいと思ってます。〔このせいで〕本当に落ち込んでしまいます［精神的にも身体的にも具合が悪くなる］。
看護師：	検査は身体的な原因の究明に役立ちますが，ご存知の通り，ベインブリッジ先生は子宮の機能障害による出血かもしれないと考えています。身体的な原因は見つからないかもしれません。
H夫人：	生理痛［月経困難症］もとても苦しいです［極度の苦痛を味わっています］。若い頃に生理痛がありましたけど，今の痛みのほうはもっとつらいです。
看護師：	〔生理痛に〕何の薬を飲んでいますか？
H夫人：	ただパラセタモールですが，あまり効きません［あまり効果的ではない］。解決したいと言ったことはわかっていますが，先生が子宮摘出の必要があると言うかもしれないと不安です。

Nurse:	There are several different treatments for heavy bleeding, such as tablets, hormones and a fairly new technique called ablation, where the lining of the womb is removed. There is lots to try before hysterectomy needs to be considered.
Mrs H.:	I do hope so. You hear about women having a hysterectomy and never really getting over it [recovering], plus all those things that happen to you.
Nurse:	What sort of things?
Mrs H.:	Well you put on weight.
Nurse:	There is no reason for anyone to put on weight after a hysterectomy other than the usual reasons of eating too much and not getting enough exercise.
Mrs H.:	It wouldn't feel right somehow.
Nurse:	In what way?
Mrs H.:	You know — not feeling like a proper woman.
Nurse:	If Mr Bainbridge advised a hysterectomy and you were considering it, the usual thing would be for you to see one of us specialist nurses again to have a proper discussion about the operation before it went ahead. But we could talk it through [discuss fully] now if you would like to.
Mrs H.:	Yes please. if you've got time now.

看護師: ひどい出血にはそれぞれに異なる治療法がいくつかありますよ。例えば，錠剤，ホルモン療法。それに，アブレーションという，比較的新しい技術で，子宮の内壁を除去するものもあります。子宮摘出を検討しなければならなくなる前に，試してみることはたくさんあります。

H夫人: 本当にそう願います。子宮摘出をして，本当には立ち直っていない［回復していない］女性のことや，それに加えて，それによって起こるいろんなことを耳にします。

看護師: どんなことでしょう？

H夫人: ええっと，太るとか。

看護師: 食べ過ぎと運動不足といった普通の理由のほかは，子宮摘出後に太る理由はありませんよ。

H夫人: どうしてか，しっくりこない気がするんです。

看護師: どういう風にですか？

H夫人: あの，ちゃんとした女性でないような。

看護師: ベインブリッジ先生があなたに子宮摘出を勧めていて，あなたがそれを検討しているとしましょう。その場合は，手術の前に私たち専門看護師のうちの1人と会い，手術についてちゃんとした話し合いを持つのが普通ですよ。でも，お望みなら，今そのことについてよく話し合う［十分に議論する］こともできます。

H夫人: はい，もし今時間がおありでしたらお願いします。

Unit 13 ANXIETY, STRESS AND DEPRESSION

Some nursing/medical or Standard English words and corresponding colloquial words and expressions associated with anxiety, stress and depression are given in Box. 11.

Note: Colloquial expressions used in the case histories and example conversations are explained in brackets [...].

BOX. 11
Words associated with anxiety, stress and depression

Nursing/medical or Standard English words	Colloquial (everyday) or slang (very informal) words and expressions used by patients
Anxious	Jumpy; nervy; wired (often used in connection with substance misuse)
Depressed	Down in the dumps/mouth; feeling down; got the hump; hacked or naffed off (also means annoyed); low (Note: Many of these expressions describe mild mood change rather than a depressive illness)
Mental health problem	Barmy; batty; bonkers; cracked/crackers; crazy; cuckoo; loony; loopy; mad; mental; nuts/nutty; off one's chump[95]/head/rocker/trolley; out of one's mind; round the bend; screw loose[96]; screwy
Stressed	Strung out; up tight

Case history 19   A panic attack: Mr Reeves

Mr Reeves has always worried about things at work and often becomes anxious if he can't clear his desk each day. Recently, he doesn't seem to

---

95.chump「頭」
96.screw loose「おかしい」ねじのゆるんだ〔抜けた〕器具の連想から。

Unit 13　　　　　　　　　　　　　　　不安，ストレス，うつ

不安，ストレス，うつに関連する看護・医学用語あるいは標準英語，並びにそれと対応する口語的な用語と表現が Box. 11 にまとめられている。

注記：病歴と会話例文中における口語的な表現には，[　] 内に説明を加えた。

Box. 11
不安，ストレス，うつに関連する用語

看護／医学用語，または標準英語の用語	患者が使う口語的（日常的）または，俗語の（非常にくだけた）用語と表現
心配な	びくびくしている；びくびくしている；興奮した（しばしば薬物の乱用と関連して使われる）
落ち込んだ	落ち込んでいる；元気がない；落ち込んでいる（いらいらしている，という意味もある）；落ち込んでいる（注：これらの表現の多くは，うつ病（の症状）というより，情緒の軽い変調を表す）
精神衛生上の問題	ちょっと気のふれた；変わっている；まともじゃない；頭のおかしい／頭のおかしい；頭がおかしい；気のふれた；頭がおかしい；頭がおかしい；どうかしている；頭がおかしい；気がふれた／気がふれた；頭がおかしい／頭がおかしい／頭がおかしい／頭がおかしい；頭がどうかしている；気が変な；おかしい；気が変な
ストレスを感じた	へとへとである；神経がぴりぴりしている

症例 19　　パニック発作：リーヴズ氏

リーヴズ氏はいつも仕事のことを心配している。そして毎日机の上を整理できないと不安になることが多い。最近，彼はうまく集中することができないようで，

be able to concentrate properly and has been staying late at work to get the day's jobs finished. He has started to feel anxious about returning to work after the weekend, and on two occasions he has had a panic attack during the bus ride to work on a Monday morning.

🔵 20

Nurse:	Hello Mr Reeves. I'm Nurse Owen. Is it all right if I ask you some questions?
Mr R.:	Yes.
Nurse:	I understand that you have had some panic attacks.
Mr R.:	Yes, when I had to go back to work after the weekend.
Nurse:	Tell me what happened.
Mr R.:	It came out of the blue [suddenly, without warning]. I felt uneasy and came over [felt] all sweaty, my heart was pounding [palpitations] and my chest felt like it would burst. I thought I was about to snuff it [die].
Nurse:	What did you do?
Mr R.:	I tried to calm down and take some big breaths, but it didn't work [not effective] and I had to get off the bus in a hurry and pushed my way off. People must have thought I was round the bend [have a mental health problem].
Nurse:	Did you get to work in the end?
Mr R.:	No, I needed to get home.
Nurse:	Were things any better once you got home?
Mr R.:	The panic had gone, but I felt edgy [nervous, irritable].
Nurse:	How do you mean?
Mr R.:	I couldn't settle to anything [moved from task to task] and was fidgety [nervously touching or playing with things] all day.
Nurse:	Tell me about your job.

その日の仕事を片づけるために遅くまで残業している。週末明けに仕事に戻ることに不安を感じるようになり始め，月曜日の朝，仕事に行くバスの中で2度パニック発作を起こした。

看護師： こんにちは，リーヴズさん。看護師のオーエンです。いくつか質問してもよろしいですか？

R氏： はい。

看護師： 何度かパニック発作を起こしたそうですね。

R氏： はい，週末明けに仕事に戻らなければならなかったときです。

看護師： どうなったか教えてください。

R氏： それは思いがけず［突然，何の前触れもなく］起こりました。不安を感じて，急に汗びっしょりになり［［汗びっしょりになるのを］感じ］，心臓がドキドキして［動悸がして］，胸が張り裂けそうでした。くたばる［死ぬ］かと思いましたよ。

看護師： どうしたんですが？

R氏： 落ち着こうと，大きく深呼吸をしようとしました。でもうまくいかなかった［効果がなかった］ので，急いでバスを降りなければならず，人を押しのけました。みんな私の頭が変になった［精神衛生上の問題を抱えていた］と思ったでしょうね。

看護師： 結局仕事には行きましたか？

R氏： いいえ，家に帰らなければなりませんでした。

看護師： 家に着いたら少しは良くなりましたか？

R氏： パニックは収まりましたが，いらいらするのを感じました［神経過敏でした，怒りっぽくなっていました］。

看護師： どういう意味ですか？

R氏： 腰を落ち着けて物事をするということができなくて［しなければならないことに次から次へと手をつけて］，1日中落ち着きがありませんでした［いらいらしてものを触ったり，いじったりしていました］。

看護師： お仕事について話してください。

25	Mr R.:	I work for an insurance company in the claims department.
	Nurse:	What does that involve?
	Mr R.:	I deal with claims from clients. It's mainly people damaging things at home or perhaps they have had a break-in [burglary]. It must be dreadful and I worry about getting the claims agreed quickly if someone has had a break-in.
	Nurse:	Do your managers put pressure on you to complete claims within a set time?
	Mr R.:	Yes, it's all about targets and outcomes, but you must know. It's like that in the NHS these days[97].
35	Nurse:	Yes, most people seem to have pressures at work.
	Mr R.:	It started when I wanted be the quickest to get claims sorted out.
	Nurse:	What happened?
	Mr R.:	I was working against the clock [pushed for time] and I managed for a while, but then I felt that I must complete everything the same day.
	Nurse:	Was that realistic?
	Mr R.:	No, but I couldn't see that. I stayed most evenings, but seemed to get less and less done.
45	Nurse:	Why do you think that happened?
	Mr R.:	I couldn't concentrate and went from job to job without finishing it. I couldn't deal with claims that were anything out of the ordinary [unusual].
	Nurse:	How did you cope?
50	Mr R.:	Well I didn't cope. I just put them to the bottom of my pile of work.
	Nurse:	How has the work situation affected your daily life?
	Mr R.:	I'm finding it hard to get out of the house [leave] for work in the mornings.

---

97. It's like that in the NHS these days.「最近のNHSにおけるようなもの」NHSは財政赤字に陥り、スタッフ削減や病院の閉鎖などを行っているため、医療従事者のオーバーワークや改革に対する反発が取りざたされている。

R氏：	保険会社の請求金部署で働いています。
看護師：	どういったことをするのですか？
R氏：	顧客の保険金申請を取り扱っています。主に自宅で何かを壊した人たちです。ことによると，不法侵入にあった［強盗に入られた］人たちもいます。とてもいやなことでしょうから，不法侵入の場合は保険金申請が速やかに認められるか気になります。
看護師：	あなたの上司は設定時間内に保険金申請を完了するようプレッシャーをかけてきますか？
R氏：	はい，目標と成果がすべてです。でも，あなたにはわかりますよね。最近のNHSのようなものです。
看護師：	そうですね，たくさんの人が仕事でプレッシャーを抱えているようですね。
R氏：	保険金申請の処理を1番早く終わらせたいと思ったときから始まりました。
看護師：	どうなったんですか？
R氏：	時間を気にしながら［時間がなくて困りながら］働きました。しばらくはどうにかしていましたが，それから，1日のうちにすべて終わらせなければと感じました。
看護師：	それは現実的でしたか？
R氏：	いいえ，でも，それがわからなかったんです。ほとんど毎晩残業しましたが，処理できる量はどんどん少なくなっていったようでした。
看護師：	どうしてそんなことになったと思いますか？
R氏：	集中できなくて，終わらせることなく次々に違う仕事に手をつけていったんです。普通ではない［珍しい］保険金申請はどれも扱えませんでした。
看護師：	どう対処しましたか？
R氏：	いえ，処理しませんでした。ただ山積みの仕事の中の1番後ろに回しただけです。
看護師：	仕事の状況で日常生活にどんな影響がありますか？
R氏：	朝，出勤で家を出る［出かける］のがつらいです。

	Nurse:	Anything else?
	Mr R.:	Same sort of problems as the ones at work. I can't concentrate on one thing and keep starting things and then leaving it to start something else. Doing the shopping is a nightmare [in this context means 'an ordeal']. I just wander from aisle to aisle picking items up and putting them down. It takes me over an hour and then I forget lots of items.
	Nurse:	Do you feel under stress?
	Mr R.:	Most of the time.
	Nurse:	What sort of things make you feel stressed?
	Mr R.:	Work obviously, but things at home can hassle me [in this context means 'worry'] as well.
	Nurse:	At home [in this context reflecting what Mr Reeves has said]?
	Mr R.:	Yes, paying bills on time and the state of the garden, it's like a jungle [very untidy]. When I feel uptight [stressed] I get really fussy about piddling [petty, unimportant] things that don't matter.
	Nurse:	What do you normally do to relieve the stress?
	Mr R.:	Listening to music helps and I've started doing yoga again.
	Nurse:	Your GP [general practitioner] thought that our team might be able to offer you some help.
	Mr R.:	Yes, we discussed some of the options, but I need more details.

Case history 20   Worries at school: Mel

Mel, aged 16 years, has just started at a new school. She had to change schools when her parents split up [divorced]. It has been difficult to make new friends and she is worried about the exams in the summer.

看護師：	ほかにはありますか？
R氏：	職場と同じ種類の問題です。1つのことに集中できず，何かを始めては，ほかの何かを始めるためにそれを放置する，ということを繰り返すのです。買い物は悪夢［この文脈では「苦しい体験」を意味する］です。ただ通路から通路をうろうろして，品物を手に取っては置くんです。1時間以上もかかるのに，買い忘れがたくさんあります。
看護師：	ストレスを感じますか？
R氏：	ほとんどいつも〔感じています〕。
看護師：	どういった事柄にストレスを感じますか？
R氏：	明らかに仕事ですが，家のことで面倒だと感じることもあります［この文脈では，「苦しい」を意味する］。
看護師：	家で？［この文脈では，リーヴズさんが言ったことを受けて］
R氏：	はい，請求書の代金を期限通りに支払うことや，庭の状態などです。まるでジャングルみたいになっています［とても見苦しいです］。ピリピリして［ストレスを感じて］いるときには，たいしたことではない，つまらない［ささいな，重要ではない］ことがとても気になります。
看護師：	ストレス解消のために普段することは何ですか？
R氏：	音楽を聴くのは役に立ちます，それから，またヨガを始めました。
看護師：	かかりつけのGP［一般開業医］は私たちのチームが何かお役に立てるのではと考えていますね。
R氏：	はい，私たちは選択肢のいくつかについて話し合いましたが，もっと詳しく知りたいんです。

症例20　　学校での心配ごと：メル

16歳のメルは，新しい学校に通い始めたばかりである。彼女は両親が別れた［離婚した］とき，転校しなければならなかった。新しい友達を作るのは難しく，夏の試験について心配している。

Nurse:	Hello, I'm Nurse Sanchez. May I call you Mel?
Mel:	If you like.
Nurse:	What would you like to talk to me about?
Mel:	You know, I moved here last term when my mum [mother] and dad [father] split up [divorced].
Nurse:	Yes, you came from St. Mary's didn't you?
Mel:	Yeah [yes], it was cool [OK, excellent] there.
Nurse:	How are you settling in here?
Mel:	Don't know really.
Nurse:	What about the people in your class? Have you made any friends?
Mel:	They've all known each other since year 7 [the first year in high school]. They don't want me — they think I'm stupid.
Nurse:	Is that what you think?
Mel:	Yeah, 'cos [because] of the row [quarrel] I had with that girl who's always talking.
Nurse:	How do you feel about the quarrel?
Mel:	It's getting me down [depressing me].
Nurse:	Have you felt like crying at all?
Mel:	I'm usually OK, as long as [provided] they don't keep picking on [bully, tease] me. During PE [physical education] I burst into tears when they made a thing about not picking me [choosing me] for their team. They said I was naff [in this context means 'useless'] at sport.
Nurse:	Do feel like breaking down [bursting into tears] at other times?
Mel:	Yeah, sometimes at home for no reason, but my mum [mother] says I should try not to take things to heart [try not to be too hurt by people's remarks].

看護師：	こんにちは。**看護師のサンチェス**です。あなたのことをメルと呼んでもいいですか？
メル：	どうぞ。
看護師：	どんなことについて話がしたいですか？
メル：	ママ［母親］とパパ［父親］が別れて［離婚して］この前の学期にここに引っ越して来たでしょう？
看護師：	ええ，セント・メアリーズから来たんでしたね？
メル：	うん［はい］，あそこはよかったの［問題ない，すごくよかった］。
看護師：	ここには慣れてきた？
メル：	よくわからない。
看護師：	クラスの人はどう？友達はできた？
メル：	あの子たちはみんな7学年［高校1年］からずっと付き合いがあるんです。私のことは必要じゃないの — 私のことをバカだと思ってる。
看護師：	そんな風に思うの？
メル：	ええ，だって［'cos は because「なぜなら」の略］いつもおしゃべりする女の子と口げんか［口論］をしたから。
看護師：	言い争いについてはどんな風に思ってるの？
メル：	落ち込んでます［気がめいります］。
看護師：	少しでも泣きたくなったはことある？
メル：	いつもは大丈夫です。あの子たちが私をいじめ［いじめ，からかい］続けなければ［続けない限りは］。PE［体育］の授業中，その子たちが私を一緒のチームに入れない［選ばない］ことで大騒ぎしたときはすごく泣いてしまったけど。私のことをスポーツでつかえない［この文脈では，「役に立たない」］って言ってた。
看護師：	ほかのときで泣き出したくなった［大泣きしたくなった］ことはある？
メル：	うん，家にいるときに，たまにわけもなく。でも，ママ［母親］は気にしないように［人の言葉であんまり傷つかないように］しなさいと言います。

	Nurse:	Did you tell your mum that you just felt like crying?
30	Mel:	I don't want to worry her. She's having a bad time.
	Nurse:	Because of the divorce?
	Mel:	Yeah, she was gutted [very upset].
	Nurse:	How have you been feeling generally?
35	Mel:	Sort of sad and fed up [bored, discontented].
	Nurse:	Are you able to enjoy the things you used to do?
	Mel:	I can't be bothered to get dolled up [get dressed up]. You can't go out on your own.
	Nurse:	What about hobbies?
40	Mel:	I used to help out at the local riding stables[98].
	Nurse:	Yes?
	Mel:	I gave it up [stopped] when we moved to this place. I can't get interested in anything now.
45	Nurse:	Apart from what you have told me is there anything else you are particularly worried about?
	Mel:	Yeah, I'm frantic [very worried] about my exams.
	Nurse:	What are you planning to do [career plans, etc.]?
	Mel:	Yeah, I really want to go to uni' [university] to do law, so I need good grades.
50	Nurse:	It's difficult changing schools just before exams.
	Mel:	Tell me about it [in this context, emphasises that Mel knows this already].
	Nurse:	How is your studying going?
55	Mel:	I should do a plan, but I keep putting it off [delaying]. It's easier to watch TV [television].
	Nurse:	How are you sleeping?
	Mel:	It's difficult to drop off [get to sleep] worrying about my revision.
	Nurse:	What about your appetite?
60	Mel:	OK, if you count junk food. If my mum is out I just have

98.riding stables「乗用馬厩舎」時間単位で馬をレンタルしてくれる。

看護師：	お母さんに泣きたくなったことを言った？
メル：	お母さんを心配させたくない。つらい思いをしているの。
看護師：	離婚のせいで？
メル：	うん，お母さんはがっくりしてた［とても動揺してた］。
看護師：	いつもは大体どんな気分がする？
メル：	なんとなく悲しくて，うんざりする［退屈している，不満がある］。
看護師：	以前楽しんでいたことを今でも楽しめる？
メル：	わざわざおしゃれする［着飾る］気になれなくて。1人では出かけられないでしょ。
看護師：	趣味はどう？
メル：	前は地元の乗用馬厩舎で手伝いをしてました。
看護師：	そうなの？
メル：	ここに引っ越してきたときにやめました［おしまいにしました］。今は興味を持てるものが何もなくて。
看護師：	今まで話してくれたこととは別に，何か特に心配なことはある？
メル：	うん，おかしくなりそうなほど試験が気になる［とても心配］。
看護師：	これから何をしようと思ってるの［キャリア・プランなど］？
メル：	うーん，法律を勉強するために本当に大学［uni' は university「大学」の略］に行きたいの。だからいい成績を取らないと。
看護師：	試験の直前に転校なんて大変ね。
メル：	まったく［この文脈では，メルがこのことをすでにわかっているということを強調している］。
看護師：	勉強の進み具合はどう？
メル：	計画を立てないといけないんだけど，ずっと先延ばしに［延期］してます。TV［テレビ］を見る方が楽で。
看護師：	睡眠はどう？
メル：	復習のことが心配で，なかなか眠れません［寝つくことができません］。
看護師：	食欲は？
メル：	まあまあ。ジャンクフードも含めればだけど。ママがいないときは，フライドポテトを食べるだけです。

	chips[99].
Nurse:	When you feel sad do you ever feel like harming yourself?
Mel:	No, not really. I know my mum needs me and I'm set on [determined] being a lawyer.
Nurse:	Do you think you could talk to your mum about how you're feeling?
Mel:	I suppose it would be best.
Nurse:	The doctor might be able to help as well.
Mel:	Yeah, thanks.

---

99. chips「フライドポテト」アメリカ英語では chips は薄くスライスしたじゃがいもを揚げたものを意味するが，英国英語では厚く切ったじゃがいもを揚げたものを意味する。

看護師：	悲しい気持ちになったとき，自分を傷つけようと思ったことはある？
メル：	ううん，特には。ママが私のことを必要なのはわかってるし，弁護士になると決めて［決意して］るの。
看護師：	あなたがどういう風に感じているかお母さんに話せる？
メル：	それが1番いいだろうと思います。
看護師：	医師も助けになることがあるかもしれませんよ。
メル：	ええ，ありがとう。

Unit 14 DEMENTIA AND CONFUSION

Some nursing/medical or Standard English words and corresponding colloquial words and expressions associated with dementia and confusion are given in Box. 12.

Note: Colloquial expressions used in the case histories and example conversations are explained in brackets [...].

BOX. 12
Words associated with dementia and confusion

Nursing/medical or Standard English words	Colloquial (everyday) or slang (very informal) words and expressions used by patients
Confused	At a loss; at sea; at sixes and sevens; befuddled; bewildered; mixed up; muddled; muzzy; not with it
Demented	Crack brained; crazed; crazy; daft; dotty; non-compos mentis

Case history 21   A wife whose husband has severe dementia: Mrs Georges

Mrs Georges has cared for her husband for over a year. His condition has deteriorated rapidly and he has now been admitted to a nursing home. He has severe dementia due to Alzheimer's disease, and it is impossible for his wife to manage with him at home.

22

Mrs G.: Hello Nurse. My husband seems quite settled now. Would you like me to answer those questions?
Nurse: Hello. Yes, now's a good time. Tea will be here in half an hour [30 minutes] or so. Will you be staying to have tea with Mr Georges?

Unit 14　　　　　　　　　　　　　認知症と錯乱状態

認知症と錯乱に関連する看護・医学あるいは標準英語，並びにそれと対応する口語的な用語と表現が Box. 12 にまとめられている。

注記：病歴と会話例文中における口語的な表現には，〔　〕内に説明を加えた。

Box. 12

認知症と錯乱に関連する用語

看護／医学用語， または標準英語の用語	患者が使う口語的（日常的） または，俗語の（非常にくだけた）用語と表現
錯乱した	当惑して；途方に暮れて；混乱して；当惑して；途方に暮れた；混乱した；混乱した；ぼんやりした；飲み込めていない
認知症になった	頭が変な；錯乱した；正気でない；正気でない；頭がおかしい；心神喪失の〔ラテン語〕

症例 21　　　認知症の夫を持つ妻：ジョージズ夫人

ジョージズ夫人は 1 年以上夫の介護をしてきた。彼の症状は急速に悪化しており，今はナーシング・ホームに入所することになった。彼はアルツハイマー病で重い認知症を患っており，妻が自宅で彼の世話をするのは不可能である。

G 夫人：　こんにちは，看護師さん。夫は今かなり落ち着いているようです。質問にお答えましょうか？

看護師：　こんにちは。ええ，今がちょうどいいですね。30 分〔30 分〕かそこらでお茶が来ます。ジョージズさんとお茶を飲んでいかれますか？

	Mrs G.:	Yes, that would be nice. It's a real treat [pleasure] to sit down and have a meal that someone else has got ready.
	Nurse:	Being the only carer is such hard work.
	Mrs G.:	At home he [her husband] wouldn't let me out of his sight for a minute. You can imagine how hard it is to get a meal.
	Nurse:	Yes, how are you feeling now that Mr Georges is here with us?
	Mrs G.:	I know it was the right decision and I had it all out [discussed it fully] with the people from the Social [social workers], but I'll miss him not being at home. It had to happen. I'm completely done in [exhausted or worn-out].
	Nurse:	Tell me about Mr Georges.
	Mrs G.:	I wish you could have seen him before all this happened. He was so on the ball [alert] and always helping people. He was in the merchant navy and spent months away, so I was used to being on my own before he retired.
	Nurse:	Have you got family nearby?
	Mrs G.:	I won't be lonely. Our lad [son] lives just around the corner. I really lost my Bob [Mr Georges] when his mind started to go.
	Nurse:	When did you first notice?
	Mrs G.:	Hard to say [difficult], I suppose you expect your memory to get worse, so you put the little lapses down to [caused by] him getting older.
	Nurse:	Well we all lose our glasses and forget names.
	Mrs G.:	Yes, but it was more than that. He seemed muddled [confused] by everyday things like making a pot of tea. He would put the teabags in the kettle or make the tea with cold water.

G夫人： はい，いいですね。腰かけて，だれかに用意してもらった食事をいただくのは本当にうれしいこと［喜び］です。

看護師： たった1人での介護は本当に大変な仕事です。

G夫人： 家では彼［彼女の夫］は一瞬たりとも私を彼の見えない所へ行かせてくれませんでした。食事を準備するのがどんなに大変か想像できるでしょう。

看護師： もちろんです，ジョージズさんがここで私たちと一緒に暮らすことについて今どういうお気持ちですか？

G夫人： それは正しい決断で，福祉の人たち［ソーシャル・ワーカーたち］と十分に話し合った［十分に議論した］ことはわかっていても，夫が家にいないと寂しくなると思います。起こるべくして起こったことなのですが。私は完全に疲れ切って［疲労困憊して，疲れ果てて］しまっていて。

看護師： ジョージズさんのことを教えてください。

G夫人： こんなことがいろいろと起こる前に，あなたが彼に会えていたらと思います。とてもてきぱきしていて［頭の回転が速くて］いつも人助けをしていました。商船の船乗りで，何か月も留守にしたもので，彼が退職するまで，私は1人でいることに慣れていました。

看護師： 近くにご家族はいらっしゃいますか？

G夫人： 1人ぼっちになることはありません。子供［息子］がすぐ近くに住んでいます。私は，ボブ［ジョージズ氏］が精神的に衰えてきたときに，実際に「私のボブ」を失ったんです。

看護師： 最初に気がついたのはいつですか？

G夫人： よくわからないんです［難しいです］，記憶力が悪くなるのは当然だと思うでしょう，だから，ふとした間違いは彼が年を取ってきているせいだと［それによって引き起こされていると］思っていました。

看護師： ええ，だれでも眼鏡を失くしたり，名前を忘れたりしますよね。

G夫人： はい，でも，それだけではありませんでした。彼はポット1杯のお茶を淹れるといった，日常的な事柄にもまごつく［混乱する］ようでした。よくティーバッグをヤカンに入れたり，冷水でお茶を淹れたりしていました。

35	Nurse:	How was he in himself?
	Mrs G.:	At first he knew something was wrong. He was frustrated and would fly off the handle [be irritable] with me and I would snap back. I didn't realise he couldn't help it [not his fault].
40	Nurse:	How do you feel about it now?
	Mrs G.:	Real bad. I feel weepy [tearful] just talking about it. Silly isn't it?
	Nurse:	No it's not silly, not at all.
	Mrs G.:	After 40 years married we knew what the other was thinking most of the time and now we're not even on the same wavelength[100] [don't understand one another].
	Nurse:	What other things have been happening?
	Mrs G.:	He would witter on and on [go on] about the same thing and asking me the same question. I'd say to him 'Bob you're driving me up the wall [irritating me]', he'd smile and next minute do it again. But he hardly says a word now [does not speak very much].
	Nurse:	What about washing and dressing?
	Mrs G.:	Gets in a right[101] pickle[102] [difficulty] with dressing. I have to help him. It's as if he can't remember what to do. Getting him to shave is a right carry-on [performance], he just won't do it and pushes me away if I try to help. I hate to see him so scruffy [untidy]. He was always so particular with his turn out [clothes and appearance]. I don't know whether you'll have better luck with him.
	Nurse:	The care assistants have special training sessions and they're all used to looking after people who have problems like Mr Georges'.
	Mrs G.:	But they won't know how to stop him getting in a lather

---

100. wavelength「個人の物の考え方, 波長」
101. right「(悪いものについて) 本当の, まったくの」
102. pickle「困った状態」

看護師：	彼自身はどうでしたか？
G夫人：	最初は，何かがおかしいと彼はわかっていました。ストレスを感じて，急に怒ったりして［怒りっぽくなって］，私もきつく言い返していました。彼にはどうしようもなかった［彼のせいではなかった］のがわからなかったんです。
看護師：	今はどういうお気持ちですか？
G夫人：	本当にひどいです。そのことを話しているだけで泣きたく［涙が出そうに］なります。ばかばかしいでしょ？
看護師：	いいえ，まったくばかばかしくなんてないですよ。
G夫人：	40年間結婚していて，ほとんどいつもお互いが何を考えているかわかっていました。今では波長が合いさえしません［お互いに理解していません］。
看護師：	ほかにどういうことがありましたか？
G夫人：	彼はくだらない，同じことをいつまでも話し続けて［しゃべり続けて］，私に同じことを質問し続けました。「ボブ，あなたのせいで頭がおかしくなりそう［いらいらする］」と言うと，彼はニッコリして，次の瞬間また同じことを繰り返してました。でも，今では彼はほとんど一言も話しません［あまりしゃべりません］。
看護師：	体を洗ったり，身支度をするのはどうですか？
G夫人：	身支度には本当に手を焼きます［は大変です］。手伝わなければなりません。まるで，彼は何をしたらいいのか思い出せないみたいなんです。髭剃りをさせるのはまったくの大騒ぎ［大変なこと］で，自分ではしようとしないし，手伝おうとすると私を押しのけます。彼のこんなに見苦しい［だらしがない］姿を見なければならないのは本当に嫌です。いつでも自分の身なり［服と外見］にはとてもうるさい人でしたから。ここのほうが彼とうまくいくかどうかはわかりません。
看護師：	介護士は特別な研修を受けていますし，みんなジョージズさんと似たような問題を抱えている人を世話するのに慣れていますよ。
G夫人：	でも，どうやって彼が興奮［動揺］するのを止めるかわからないでしょう？

Nurse: [agitated].

Nurse: Would you like to meet the team who will be caring for Mr Georges, so you can tell them about the best way to do things? Most relatives say it's reassuring.

Mrs G.: That would put my mind at rest [feel reassured] about leaving him here. I will just say that he seems to like sitting in front of the box[103] [television]. He can't know what's on but he does seem calmer. Before he got this bad he was forever changing channels and I never got to see the end of anything.

Nurse: How frustrating for you. Does Mr Georges wander about?

Mrs G.: In the last few months it started. He kept wandering off during the day. He was off like a shot [moved quickly] and he'd be in the road before I got out the house. I was sure he'd be under a car at any moment [have a road accident]. And then he stopped knowing day and night and would get up [out of bed] at all hours of the night. That really scared me. What if he'd turned on the gas [the gas cooker/oven]? He was always fiddling [touching] with it during the day.

Nurse: That must have been a real worry.

Mrs G.: I'd lay there in the dark listening for him getting up, and when I dropped off [got to sleep] any little noise would wake me. That's what really decided me about him coming here.

Nurse: I just heard the tea trolley go by. We can finish this later if you like.

Mrs G.: I could do with a cuppa [usually refers to a cup of tea] I'm parched [thirsty].

---

103. box「テレビ」英国口語。

| 看護師： | ジョージズさんの介護にあたるチームとお会いになりませんか？〔世話をするのに〕1番良い方法を彼らに伝えられます。たいていの親類の方が心強く感じられると言いますよ。 |

G夫人： そうすれば，彼をここに預けても安心です［安心します］。彼はTV［テレビ］の前に座るのが好きなようだとだけお伝えしましょう。〔テレビで〕何をやっているかはわかっていないけれど，ずっと落ち着いて見えることは確かです。これほどひどくなる前は，ちょこちょことチャンネルを変えてしまって，私はどれも終わりまで見られませんでした。

看護師： それはいらいらしたでしょう。ジョージズさんに徘徊はありますか？

G夫人： この2, 3か月で始まりました。日中，彼はずっとうろうろしていました。飛んで行って［素早く移動して］，私が家を出る前に道路に出てしまうのです。いつ車の下にいても［交通事故にあっても］おかしくないと思いました。それから，彼は昼と夜の区別がつかなくなり，夜中じゅうずっと起きて［ベッドから出て］いました。もし，彼がガス［ガスレンジ／オーブン］のスイッチを入れたらどうしよう，と本当に怖かったです。日中ずっといじって［触って］いたものですから。

看護師： 本当に心配だったでしょう。

G夫人： 暗闇の中で横になって，彼が起き上がる音に聞き耳を立てていました。うとうとしていても［寝たときでも］，どんな小さな音にも目が覚めました。実際，それで彼をここに連れてこようと決心したのです。

看護師： たった今お茶のワゴンが通る音が聞こえました。よろしければ，話の続きは後にしましょう。

G夫人： 1杯［通常お茶1杯を指す］あればありがたいです。喉がからからです［渇いています］。

Unit 15 PAIN

Some nursing/medical or Standard English words and corresponding colloquial words and expressions associated with pain are given in Box. 13.

Note: Colloquial expressions used in the case histories and example conversations are explained in brackets [...].

BOX. 13

Words associated with pain

Nursing/medical or Standard English words	Colloquial (everyday) or slang (very informal) words and expressions used by patients
Analgesic	Painkiller
Grimaces	Pull a face
Pain	Ache; agony; cramp; discomfort; hurt; irritation; smarting; soreness; spasm; tenderness; throb; twinge (see text for more words used to describe pain)

'Pain' and 'ache' mean the same thing and we speak of 'aches and pains' generally. Both these words are nouns, but the word 'ache' can be used with the following to form a compound noun: backache, earache, headache, stomach-ache (usually means an ache in the abdomen), toothache. For the other parts of the body, we say:

'I have a pain in my shoulder, chest, etc.'

It is possible to have a pain in the back, head and stomach (usually means the abdomen), but this generally refers to a more serious condition than backache, headache and stomach-ache.

The word 'ache' can also be used as a verb:

'My leg aches after walking 10 miles.'
'My back aches after gardening.'

Unit 15   痛み

痛みに関連する看護・医学用語あるいは標準英語,並びにそれと対応する口語的な用語と表現が Box. 13 にまとめられている。

注記：病歴と会話例文中における口語的な表現には，〔　〕内に説明を加えた。

BOX. 13
痛みに関連する単語

看護／医学用語，または標準英語の用語	患者が使う口語的 (日常的) または，俗語の (非常にくだけた) 用語と表現
鎮痛薬	痛み止め
しかめ面	しかめ顔をする
痛み	痛み；激痛；けいれん；不快感；苦痛；炎症；ひりひり痛むこと；〔触れた際の〕痛み；筋肉のけいれん圧痛；ずきずき痛むこと；激痛（痛みを表すのに用いられる，さらに多くの単語については本文を参照）

痛みを表す pain と ache は同じ意味で，一般的に，aches and pains〔ある一定の間続く軽い痛み〕という表現が使われる。この単語は両者とも名詞だが，ache という単語は次のように複合名詞を形成するのに用いることができる：backache「背中の痛み，腰痛」, earache「耳痛」, headache「頭痛」, stomach-ache「胃痛，通常お腹の痛みを意味する」, toothache「歯痛」。体のほかの部分に関しては，次のように表す：

　　「肩，胸，などに痛みがある」

背中，頭，そして胃（通常お腹を意味する）に have a pain を使うことは可能だが，一般的に，ache の複合語，backache「背中の痛み」, headache「頭痛」, そして stomach-ahce「胃痛」よりも深刻な症状を指す。

ache という単語は動詞としても使うことができる。

　　「10 マイル歩いたので脚が痛む。」
　　「庭いじりをしたので背中〔腰〕が痛む。」

The word 'hurt' is another verb used to express injury and pain:

> 'My chest hurts when I cough.'
> 'My neck hurts when I turn my head.'

How patients describe pain: commonly used words

—aching
—beating
—biting
—boring
—burning (as in cystitis, oesophagitis)
—bursting
—colicky (often used to describe the pain that results from periodic spasm in an abdominal organ (biliary, intestinal), but also used to describe renal colic and dysmenorrhoea)
—crampy
—crushing (as in angina pectoris or myocardial infarction)
—cutting (rectal disease)
—discomfort (may describe mild pain sensation)
—dragging (as in uterine prolapse)
—drawing
—dull (headache, tumour)
—gnawing (tumour) (pronounced nawing)
—grinding
—griping
—gripping (as in angina pectoris)
—heavy (as pre-menstrual)
—knife-like
—numb (lack of sensation)

hurt という単語は怪我や痛みを表現する別の動詞である。

「咳をすると胸が痛む。」
「頭の向きを変えると首が痛む。」

患者がどのように痛みを表現するか：一般的に使われる単語

〔　〕内は訳者補足

- aching　　　　痛い
- beating　　　　ずきずきする
- biting　　　　ひりひりする
- boring　　　　〔痛みが〕突き刺すような
- burning　　　　やけるような（膀胱炎，食道炎で見られるような）
- bursting　　　　破裂するような，張り裂けるような
- colicky　　　　疝痛の（腹部の臓器《胆管，腸》の周期的なけいれんから生じる痛みを表すのにしばしば用いられるが，腎疝痛や月経困難を表すのにも用いられる）
- crampy　　　　けいれん性の〔差し込むような〕
- crushing　　　　圧迫されるような〔押しつぶされるような〕（狭心症や心筋梗塞でみられる）
- cutting　　　　切るような（直腸の病気）
- discomfort　　　　不快感のある（軽い痛みの感覚を表すこともある）
- dragging　　　　牽引〔性〕の〔引っ張られるような〕（子宮脱に見られるような）
- drawing　　　　引っ張られるような
- dull　　　　鈍い（頭痛，腫瘍）
- gnawing　　　　しつこい〔しくしく痛む，さしこむ〕（腫瘍）（[nɔːiŋ] と発音）
- grinding　　　　しくしく痛む〔さしこむ，きりきり痛む，じりじり痛む〕
- griping　　　　きりきり痛む
- gripping　　　　わしづかみにされるような（狭心症に見られるような）
- heavy　　　　だるい〔鈍い〕（月経前に見られるような）
- knife-like　　　　〔痛みが〕切られたような
- numb　　　　無感覚の〔麻痺した，しびれた〕（無感覚）

- piercing (angina pectoris)
- pinching
- pounding (headache - 'My head is pounding')
- pressing
- prickling (as in conjunctivitis)
- scalding (cystitis)
- severe pain (gip — 'It gives me the gip')
- sharp
- shooting (sciatica, toothache)
- sickening
- smarting (burns)
- sore
- spiky
- splinter-like
- stabbing (indigestion)
- stinging (cuts, stings)
- stitch (sudden sharp pain usually due to spasm of the diaphragm)
- straining
- tearing
- tender
- throbbing (headache, an infected area)
- tingling (return of circulation to extremities)
- twinge (sudden, sharp)
- twisting.

Pain may also be described as being: acute, agonising, chronic, constant, constricting, convulsive, darting, deep-seated, difficult to move, diffuse, excruciating, fleeting, intense, intermittent, localised, mild, obstinate, persistent, radiating, severe, spasmodic, spreading, stubborn, superficial, very severe, violent.

— piercing	刺すような（狭心症）	
— pinching	つねられるような〔締めつけるような，圧迫するような〕	
— pounding	ズキズキ〔ガンガン〕する（頭痛 —「頭がズキズキする」）	
— pressing	押しつけるような〔圧迫するような，締めつけるような〕	
— prickling	チクチクする（結膜炎に見られるような）	
— scalding	〔痛みが〕やけどしているような（膀胱炎）	
— severe pain	激痛（〔俗語で〕gip とも —「激痛がする」）	
— sharp	鋭い，激しい	
— shooting	〔痛みが〕刺すような（坐骨神経痛，歯痛）	
— sickening	吐き気〔不快感〕を引き起こすような	
— smarting	ズキズキする〔ひりひりする〕（やけど）	
— sore	ヒリヒリする	
— spiky	〔間隔をおいて〕鋭く痛む	
— splinter-like	バラバラになるような〔裂けたような〕	
— stabbing	突き刺すような（消化不良）	
— stinging	チクチクする（切り傷，刺し傷）	
— stitch	わき腹の痛み〔差し込み〕（通常横隔膜のけいれんのために生じる突然の鋭い痛み）	
— straining	引き違えた〔くじいた〕	
— tearing	引き裂くような〔かきむしるような〕	
— tender	触ると痛い	
— throbbing	ズキズキする（頭痛，感染した場所）	
— tingling	刺痛〔しびれ感，ピリピリ感〕（血液の循環が四肢に戻ってくる）	
— twinge	激痛〔刺痛〕（急な，鋭い）	
— twisting.	ねじれたような〔よじれるような〕	

痛みは次のように表すこともできる：急性の〔激しい〕，大変に激しい，慢性の，持続する，締めつけられるような，けいれん性の〔発作的な〕，ずきずきする，深在性の，動かしづらい，広範性の，耐え難い，一瞬の，激しい，断続的な，局部的な，軽度の，難治性〔しつこい〕，持続性の，放散する，ひどい，けいれん性の，拡散する，しぶとい，表面の，とてもひどい，猛烈な。

Case history 22   Migraine attacks: Miss Carter

Miss Carter has had migraine attacks for many years, but recently they are coming more often and her usual tablets are not as effective. This has led to her having several days off sick from work.

🔊 23

Miss C.: My heads [in this context meaning the 'migraine attacks'] are getting worse. I wish I knew what brings it on [causes it].

Nurse: When did you start having migraine?

Miss C.: Oh, years ago when I was still at school, but now they're coming every couple of weeks.

Nurse: How does that differ from before?

Miss C.: I only had them once in a blue moon [very infrequently], but always when I was planning to do something special.

Nurse: Can you think of any reasons why they're coming more often?

Miss C.: Well, I've got a new job and it's more stressful.

Nurse: Can you do anything about that?

Miss C.: No chance at the moment.

Nurse: What about things like certain foods, or drinks [in this context alcoholic drinks]. Have you noticed any link?

Miss C.: I know to layoff [give up] chocolate. But now it's really spooky [weird, strange]. Sometimes I have a sip[104] of wine and my head feels tight and I just know that a migraine is on its way [going to occur], and other times I have two or three glasses and get away with it [escape having a migraine attack].

Nurse: Is it a particular type of wine?

Miss C.: No, sometimes red and sometimes white wine.

---

104. sip「一口、ひとすすり」

症例 22　　偏頭痛発作：カーターさん

カーターさんは何年も偏頭痛発作を抱えているが，最近では発作がより頻繁に起こるようになり，いつも飲んでいる錠剤が効かなくなっている。このせいで彼女は何日か仕事を病欠している。

Cさん：　頭［この文脈では，「偏頭痛の発作」を意味する］が悪化しています。どうして起こるのか［原因が］わかればいいのですが。

看護師：　偏頭痛が始まったのはいつですか？

Cさん：　ああ，まだ学生だった，もう何年も前のころです。でも，今は 2, 3 週間ごとに起こります。

看護師：　以前とどのような点が違いますか？

Cさん：　めったに［ごくまれにしか］起こらなかったのですが，いつも何か特別なことをやろうとしたときでした。

看護師：　どうして偏頭痛が前より頻繁になったか，思い当たることはありますか？

Cさん：　ええっと，新しい仕事を始めたのですが，それが前よりストレスのたまるものです。

看護師：　何か〔変更は〕できますか？

Cさん：　今のところ，可能性はありません。

看護師：　ある種の食べ物や飲み物［この文脈ではアルコール飲料］といったものについてはどうですか？何か関連性に気づいたことは？

Cさん：　チョコレートはよしたほうがいい［やめるべきである］のはわかっています。でも今は本当に気味が悪い［変な，おかしい］です。ワインを一口飲むと，頭が締めつけられるよう感じがして，偏頭痛が始まる［これから起こる］のがわかることがあれば，2, 3 杯を飲んでもやり過ごせる［偏頭痛の発作を免れる］こともあります。

看護師：　特定の種類のワインですか？

Cさん：　いいえ，赤ワインだったり，白ワインだったりです。

25	Nurse:	Does anything special make it worse once you've got the pain?
	Miss C.:	Yes, any bright light. You know like sunlight on water. It's no problem 'cos [because] I always have my dark glasses with me until I can get into bed.
30	Nurse:	What about the migraine attacks? Have they changed?
	Miss C.:	The throbbing is much worse. It's so bad I have to lie on the bed and try to sleep.
	Nurse:	Do you take anything for the pain?
	Miss C.:	I always used to take a painkiller [analgesic] and the pain
35		would soon go off [stop], but no joy [failure] now. Nothing seems to shift the pain [relieve the pain].
	Nurse:	Which painkillers?
	Miss C.:	Mostly Panadol [a proprietary name for paracetamol], but sometimes ibuprofen[105]. It depends on what I have with me.
40	Nurse:	Over the last few years much better drugs have become available for migraine.
	Miss C.:	Yes, I knew that, but it didn't matter while the Panadol still worked OK.

---

105. ibuprofen「イブプロフェン」非ステロイド系の解熱, 鎮痛, 抗炎症薬で, 痛みや炎症を引き起こすプロスタグランジンの生成を抑制する働きがある。

看護師：	痛みが始まってから，何か特別なことで悪化したりしますか？
Cさん：	はい，明るい光です。水に反射する太陽光のような。ベッドに入るまでずっとサングラスを持っているので['cos は because「〜なので」の略]問題はありません。
看護師：	偏頭痛の発作はどうですか？変わったことはありますか？
Cさん：	もっとひどくズキズキします。あまりにもひどくて，ベッドに横になって，眠ろうとしないとなりません。
看護師：	痛みのために何か飲んでいますか？
Cさん：	以前はいつも痛み止め[鎮痛剤]を飲んでました。それで痛みはすぐに消えて[止まって]いましたが，今ではうまくいきません[失敗しています]。痛みを取り除く[痛みを除去する]ものは何もないかのようです。
看護師：	痛み止めは何ですか？
Cさん：	だいたいは，パナドール[パラセタモールの商標名]ですが，イブプロフェンもたまに飲みます。〔そのとき〕持っている物によります。
看護師：	ここ数年の間に，ずっと良い薬が偏頭痛に使用できるようになりましたよ。
Cさん：	はい，それは知っていました。でも，パナドールが効いていたうちは気にかけませんでした。

THINKING ABOUT (REFLECTION) PRACTICE: EXERCISE

Think about a recent time at work when you needed to get information, or help patients/clients/relatives to understand something to do with their care.

— Who was the person?
— What did you need to find out or tell them?
— How did you start the conversation?
— Did you get the information you needed, or were you successful in helping the person understand something?
— Did you have any difficulty understanding everything the Patient / client /relative said to you?
— Do you think that they understood everything you said?
— Which parts of the communication were good and what helped to make it so?
— Which parts were less successful and what stopped them working so well?

Consider the answers you have given and pick out what you have learned from this situation. What, if anything, would you do differently if the same sort of situation happened again?

実践について考える(振り返り):問題

最近,職場で情報収集が必要だったときのことや,患者/クライエント/親戚の看護への理解を促す必要があったときについて思い出そう。

— その人はだれだったか?
— 何を知る必要があったのか,また,相手に何を伝える必要があったのか?
— どのように会話を始めたか?
— 必要な情報は得られたか,または,ちゃんと相手が何かを理解する手助けができたか?
— 患者/クライエント/親戚が言ったことすべてを理解するのに苦労したか?
— 彼らに言ったことすべてが理解されたと思うか?
— コミュニケーションのどの部分が良かったか,そして,何がそうなる助けとなったか?
— どの部分がよりうまくいかなかったか,そして,何がうまくいくのを妨げたのか?

あなたがした答えを良く考えて,この状況から学んだことを見つけ出しなさい。もし同じ種類の状況に遭遇したら,むしろ,どのように異なって対処するのだろう?

FURTHER READING

Holland K, Jenkins J, Solomon J, Whittam S 2003 Applying the Roper-Lagan-Tierney model in practice. Churchill Livingstone, Edinburgh.

Roper N, Logan WW, Tierney AJ 1996 The elements of nursing, 4th edn. Churchill Livingstone, Edinburgh.

Holland K, Jenkins J, Solomon J, Whittam S 2003 Applying the Roper-Lagan-Tierney model in practice. Churchill Livingstone, Edinburgh.

Roper N, Logan WW, Tierney AJ 1996 The elements of nursing, 4th edn. Churchill Livingstone, Edinburgh.

II GLOSSARY OF MEDICAL AND COLLOQUIAL NAMES

Medical name	Colloquial name
Alopecia	baldness
Arteriosclerosis	hardening of the arteries
Blepharitis	sore eyelids
Bursitis	housemaid's knee, tennis elbow (see epicondylitis)
Cancer	a growth, the big C, the worst, tumour
Candidiasis; monilia	thrush
Cerebral palsy	to be spastic
Cerebrovascular accident	stroke
Colic	gripes
Concussion	KO'd, to be concussed, to be knocked out
Conjunctivitis	pink eye
Contusion	bruise
Convulsions	fits
Coronary thrombosis; myocardial infarction	a coronary, heart attack
Coryza	cold
Dandruff	scurf
Delirium tremens	DTs, the jerks, the shakes
Diabetes mellitus	sugar diabetes
Dysmenorrhoea	painful periods
Dysphagia	difficulty swallowing

Ⅱ 病気の医学名と口語名の用語集

医学名	口語名
脱毛症	はげていること
動脈硬化症	動脈が硬くなること
眼瞼炎	ひりひりする瞼(まぶた)
滑液包炎	家政婦ひざ，テニスひじ（上顆炎を参照）
がん	腫瘍，がん，最悪の事態，腫瘍
カンジタ症；モニリア	鵞口瘡(がこうそう)
脳性麻痺	痙攣性の麻痺を起す
脳血管障害	脳卒中
疝痛	きりきりした痛み
脳振盪	気を失う，脳震盪を起こした，ノックアウトされた
結膜炎	はやり目
打撲傷	打撲，あざ
けいれん	ひきつけ，発作
冠状動脈血栓症；心筋梗塞	冠状動脈性心臓発作，心臓発作
鼻風邪	風邪
ふけ	ふけ
振戦せん妄	DT，せん妄症，震え
糖尿病	糖尿
月経困難症	生理痛
嚥下障害	飲み込むのが困難であること

Dyspnoea	breathless, out of breath, panting, puffed, short of breath
Dyspepsia	indigestion
Encephalitis	brain fever
Enuresis	bed-wetting
Epicondylitis	golfer's elbow (medial side), tennis elbow (lateral side)
Epistaxis	nosebleeds
Eructation	belching
Erythema pernio	chilblains
Flatulence, flatus	wind, Note: To belch (to send out wind from stomach noisily), to fart* (to send out wind from anus)
Frequency	I keep wanting to go (to pass urine)
Furuncle	boil
Gonorrhoea	clap
Haemorrhoids	piles
Halitosis	bad breath
Hernia	rupture
Herpes simplex	cold blister or sore
Herpes zoster	shingles
Hordeolum	stye
Hydrophobia	rabies
Hypertension	high blood pressure
Incontinence	leaky, not to be able to hold one's water or motions, to have an accident
Infectious mononucleosis	glandular fever
Influenza	flu

呼吸困難	息をするのが困難な，息切がする，あえぎ，息を切らして，息切れして
消化不良	消化不良
脳炎	脳炎
遺尿症	おねしょ
上顆炎（じょうかえん）	ゴルファーひじ（内側），テニスひじ（側面）
鼻出血	鼻血
おくび	げっぷ
凍傷性紅斑	しもやけ
鼓腸，腸内ガス	おなら。注：げっぷをする（音を立てて胃から空気を送り出す），おならをする（肛門から腸内のガスを送り出す）
頻度	私は何度も（排尿に）行きたくなる
フルンケル	おでき
淋病	淋病
痔核	痔
口臭	息が臭いこと
ヘルニア	ヘルニア
単純ヘルペス	単純疱疹，口唇ヘルペス
帯状疱疹	帯状疱疹
麦粒腫	物もらい
恐水症	狂犬病
高血圧	高血圧
失禁	尿を我慢できない，尿や便をこらえることができない，おもらしをする
伝染［感染］性単核球症	腺熱
インフルエンザ	インフルエンザ

Leucorrhoea	whites
Menopause	the change (of life), the turn (of life)
Menstruation	period(s)
Myopia	short-sight
Neuralgia	face ache
Nocturia	to get up at night (to pass water)
Oedema	dropsy, swelling
Osteoporosis	brittle bone disease
Parotitis (infectious)	mumps
Pediculosis capitis; head lice	nits
Peritonsillar abscess	quinsy
Pertussis	whooping cough
Poliomyelitis	infantile paralysis, polio
Pruritus	itching
Pyrexia	fever, a high temperature
Pyrosis	heartburn, water-brash
Rheumatic disease	screws, springes, rheumatics
Rubella	German measles
Rubeola; morbilli	measles
Scarlatina	scarlet fever
Seizure	convulsion, fit
Strabismus	a squint
Syncope	fainting
Tachycardia	palpitations
Tendonitis	golfer's elbow, tennis elbow
Tetanus	lockjaw

白帯下	こしけ
更年期	(人生の)変化,(人生の)変わり目
月経	生理
近視	近眼
神経痛	顔面神経痛
夜間頻尿	(排尿するために)夜間起きること
浮腫	水腫,腫れ
骨粗しょう症	骨粗しょう症
耳下腺炎(伝染性の)	おたふく風邪
頭ジラミ症;頭ジラミ	シラミ(の卵)
へんとう周囲膿瘍	へんとう腺炎
百日咳	百日咳
ポリオ	小児麻痺,ポリオ
掻痒症	かゆみ
発熱	発熱,高熱
胸焼け	胸焼け,胸焼け
リウマチ性疾患	リウマチ〔やや古い表現〕,リウマチ〔やや古い表現〕,リウマチ
風疹	風疹
麻疹,はしか	はしか
猩紅熱	猩紅熱
発作	けいれん,発作
斜視	斜視
失神	気絶すること
頻脈	動悸
腱炎	ゴルファーひじ,テニスひじ
破傷風	〔初期の〕破傷風

Tinea circinata	ringworm
Tinnitus	ringing in the ears
Tuberculosis	TB
Urticaria	heat spots, hives, nettle rash
Varicella	chickenpox
Verrucae	warts
Vesicle	blister

連環状白せん	白せん
耳鳴り	耳鳴り
結核	TB
じんましん	発疹，じんましん，発疹
水痘	水ぼうそう
いぼ	いぼ
小水疱	水膨れ

III Abbreviations used in nursing

INTRODUCTION

The rapid developments in nursing, healthcare and the related sciences in recent years have brought a vast increase in the associated vocabulary. At the same time, the increased speed of life has driven people to use abbreviations more and more, and this tendency is well illustrated in the nursing and healthcare field.

The use of abbreviations is discouraged because they are variable and misleading. The same initials may have different meanings in different areas of nursing practice. For example, PID may mean pelvic inflammatory disease or prolapsed intervertebral disc. The Nursing and Midwifery Council is clear about the need to avoid the use of abbreviations in record keeping and documentation (NMC 2002) (see Ch. 4).

Nevertheless, you will see and hear abbreviations being used every day in medical reports and notes and in discussions about patients and during handover reports, and a knowledge of them is, therefore, absolutely essential. You should always ask if you are not sure what an abbreviation means.

A selection of abbreviations commonly used by nurses and other health professionals is provided to help you understand what people mean.

A

AA — Alcoholics Anonymous
AAA — abdominal aortic aneurysm
ABG — arterial blood gas
a.c. — ante cibum (Latin sometimes used in prescriptions), before food
ACE — angiotensin-converting enzyme
ACTH — adrenocorticotrophic hormone

Ⅲ 看護で使用される略語

はじめに

近年の看護・医療と関連する科学の急速な発展により，これらに関わる語彙も膨大に増加してきている。同時に，生活の速度が速くなり，ますます略語が使われるようになってきている。この傾向は看護や医療の分野によく表れている。

変化しやすく，紛らわしいため，略語の使用は推奨されない。同じ文字でも，看護実践の異なる分野では異なる意味を持つ場合がありうるのだ。例えば，PIDは，骨盤内炎症性疾患かもしれないし，椎間板ヘルニアであるかもしれない。看護・助産師会では，記録の保管と文書の作成において略語の使用を避ける必要があることを明確にしている。（NMC 2002 年）（〔原著〕4 章〔本対訳書では省略〕参照）

それにもかかわらず，医学的報告書や文書，患者に関する議論，また申し送りにおいて略語は日常的に使われている。結局のところ，略語についての知識は必要不可欠といえる。略語が何を意味するか自信がない場合には，常に質問をするべきである。

理解の一助となるよう，看護師とその他医療専門職が広く使用している略語を精選して示す。

A

AA ― アルコホーリクス・アノニマス〔直訳すると「無名のアルコール依存症者たち」日本ではこれをもとに「断酒会」が作られた〕
AAA ― 腹部大動脈瘤
ABG ― 動脈血ガス
a.c. ― 食前（ラテン語 ― ときどき処方箋で使われる）
ACE ― アンジオテンシン変換酵素
ACTH ― 副腎皮質刺激ホルモン

ADH — antidiuretic hormone
ADHD — attention-deficit hyperactivity disorder
ad lib — ad libitum (Latin), to the desired amount
ADLs — Activities of Daily Living
ADRs — adverse drug reactions
A&E — Accident and Emergency Department
AF — atrial fibrillation
AFB — acid-fast bacilli
AFP — α-fetoprotein
AI — artificial insemination
AIDS — acquired immune deficiency syndrome
ALL — acute lymphoblastic leukaemia
ALs — Activities of Living
ALS — advanced life support
ALT — alanine aminotransferase
AMI — acute myocardial infarction
AML — acute myeloid leukaemia
ANC — antenatal care
ANS — autonomic nervous system
AP — anteroposterior
APEL — accreditation of prior experience and learning
APH — antepartum haemorrhage
APKD - adult polycystic kidney disease
ARC — AIDS-related complex
ARDS — adult respiratory distress syndrome
ARF — (1) acute renal failure; (2) acute respiratory failure
ASD — atrial septal defect

ADH — 抗利尿ホルモン

ADHD — 注意欠陥多動障害

ad lib — 適宜に，適量で（ラテン語）

ADLs — 日常生活動作

ADRs — 薬剤有害反応，副作用

A&E — 英国における「救急外来」の呼称

AF — 心房細動

AFB — 抗酸菌

AFP — アルファフェトプロテイン

AI — 人工受精

AIDS — 後天性免疫不全症候群

ALL — 急性リンパ芽球性白血病

ALs — 生活活動

ALS — 二次救命処置

ALT — アラニンアミノトランスフェラーゼ

AMI — 急性心筋梗塞

AML — 急性骨髄性白血病

ANC — 妊娠管理

ANS — 自律神経系

AP — 前後の，前後方向の

APEL — 実務経験・既習事項の単位認定制度〔成人学生のこれまでの学習経歴や，実務経験などを単位として認定する英国の大学における認定制度の1つ〕

APH — 分娩前出血

APKD — 成人型多発性囊胞腎症〔現在では ADPKD: autosomal dominant polycystic kidney disease と呼ばれることが一般的で「常染色体優性多発性囊胞腎疾患」と訳される〕

ARC — エイズ関連症候群

ARDS — 成人呼吸促迫症候群〔現在では acute respiratory distress syndrome と記載され「急性呼吸促迫症候群」と呼ばれることが一般的〕

ARF — (1) 急性腎不全；(2) 急性呼吸不全

ASD — 心房中隔欠損症

AST — aspartate aminotransferase

ATN — acute tubular necrosis

ATD — Alzheimer's-type dementia

A-V — atrioventricular: (1) node; (2) bundle

B

BAI — Beck Anxiety Inventory

BAN — British Approved Name (of drugs)

BBA — born before arrival

BBB — (1) blood-brain barrier; (2) bundle branch block

BBVs — blood-borne viruses

BCG — bacille Calmette Guérin

b.d. — bis die (Latin — sometimes used in prescriptions), twice daily

BDI — Beck Depression Inventory

BHS — Beck Hopelessness Scale

b.i.d — bis in die (Latin), twice a day

BID — brought in dead

BLS — basic life support

BMI — body mass index

BMR — basal metabolic rate

BMT — bone marrow transplant

BN — Bachelor of Nursing

BNF — British National Formulary

BNO — bowels not opened

BO — bowels opened

BP — (1) blood pressure; (2) British Pharmacopoeia

BPH — benign prostatic hyperplasia

BPRS — Brief Psychiatric Rating Scale

BSA — body surface area

BSc — Bachelor of Science

AST ― アスパラギン酸アミノトランスフェラーゼ

ATN ― 急性尿細管壊死

ATD ― アルツハイマー型認知症

A-V ― 房室の：(1) 房室結節；(2) 房室束〔「ヒス束」とも呼ばれる〕

B

BAI ― ベック不安評価尺度

BAN ― (医薬品の) 英国承認名称

BBA ― 到着前出産〔妊婦が病院に到着する前，または自宅出産において助産師が到着する前に出産すること〕

BBB ― (1) 血液脳関門；(2) 脚ブロック

BBVs ― 血液媒介ウイルス

BCG ― カルメット・ゲラン結核菌

b.d. ― 1日2回 (ラテン語 ― 処方箋でときどき使用される)

BDI ― ベックうつ病評価尺度

BHS ― ベック絶望感尺度

b.i.d ― 1日2回 (ラテン語)

BID ― 入院時死亡〔dead on arrival; DOA「来院時既死亡」と同意〕

BLS ― 一次救命処置〔心臓マッサージや人工呼吸など現場での救命行為〕

BMI ― ボディマス指数

BMR ― 基礎代謝率

BMT ― 骨髄移植

BN ― 看護学士

BNF ― 英国国立医薬品集

BNO ― 排便なし

BO ― 排便あり

BP ― (1) 血圧；(2) 英国薬局方

BPH ― 良性前立腺肥大症

BPRS ― 簡易精神医学的評価尺度，簡易精神症状評価尺度

BSA ― 体表面積

BSc ― 理学士

BSc (Soc SC-Nurs) — Bachelor of Science (Nursing)
BSE — (1) bovine spongiform encephalopathy; (2) breast self-examination
BSS — Beck Scale for Suicide Ideation
B Wt — birth weight

C

C — (1) carbon; (2) centigrade (temperature scale)
Ca — carcinoma
CABG — coronary artery bypass grafting
CAN — Camberwell Assessment of Need
CAPD — continuous ambulatory peritoneal dialysis
CAPE — Clifton Assessment Procedures for the Elderly
CATS — credit accumulation transfer scheme
cc — cubic centimetre
CCF — congestive cardiac failure
CCU — Coronary Care Unit
CD — controlled drug
CDC — Centers for Disease Control and Prevention
CDS — Calgary Depression Scale
CEA — carcinoembryonic antigen
CF — (1) cardiac failure; (2) cystic fibrosis
CHAI — Commission for Healthcare Audit and Inspection
CHD — (1) congenital heart disease; (2) coronary heart disease
CHF — congestive heart failure
CIN — cervical intraepithelial neoplasia
CINAHL — Cumulative Index to Nursing and Allied Health Literature
CJD — Creutzfeldt-Jakob disease
CK — creatine kinase
CLL — chronic lymphatic leukaemia

BSc (Soc SC-Nurs) ― 看護学士

BSE ―(1) ウシ海綿状脳症；(2) 乳房自己検診

BSS ― ベック自殺念慮評価尺度

B Wt ― 出生体重

C

C ―(1) 炭素；(2) 摂氏（温度目盛）

Ca ― 癌（がん）

CABG ― 冠動脈バイパス術

CAN ― キャンバーウェル要求度評価尺度

CAPD ― 連続携行式腹膜透析

CAPE ― クリフトン高齢者評価法〔高齢者の生活の質，身体的依存度，認識能力的依存度を測る〕

CATS ―〔学業の〕単位蓄積・互換制度

cc ― 立方センチメートル

CCF ― うっ血性心不全

CCU ― 冠〔状〕〔動脈〕疾患集中治療〔病棟〕，冠〔状〕〔動脈〕疾患〔監視〕病室

CD ― 規制薬物

CDC ― 疾病管理予防センター〔米国保健福祉省の機関〕

CDS ― カルガリーうつ病評価尺度

CEA ― 癌胎児性抗原

CF ―(1) 心不全；(2) 囊胞線維症

CHAI ― 医療監査・検査委員会〔NHS の提供する医療の適切さを監視する独立機関〕

CHD ―(1) 先天性心疾患；(2) 冠動脈性心疾患

CHF ― うっ血性心不全

CIN ― 子宮頚部上皮内腫瘍

CINAHL ― シナール〔看護と関連医療の英米の文献情報データベース〕

CJD ― クロイツフェルト・ヤコブ病

CK ― クレアチンキナーゼ

CLL ― 慢性リンパ性白血病

cm — centimetre
CML — chronic myeloid leukaemia
CMV — cytomegalovirus
CNS — (1) central nervous system; (2) clinical nurse specialist
C/O — complains of
COPD — chronic obstructive pulmonary disease
COSHH — Control of Substances Hazardous to Health
CPA — care programme approach
CPAP — continuous positive airways pressure
CPD — continuing professional development
CPN — community psychiatric nurse
CPR — cardiopulmonary resuscitation
CRF — chronic renal failure
CSCI — Commission for Social Care Inspection
CSF — (1) cerebrospinal fluid; (2) colony stimulating factor
CSI — Caregiver Strain Index
CSSD — Central Sterile Supply Department
CSU — catheter specimen of urine
CT — (1) computed tomography; (2) coronary thrombosis
CTG — cardiotocograph
CV — (1) cardiovascular; (2) curriculum vitae
CVA — cerebrovascular accident
CVP — central venous pressure
CVS — (1) cardiovascular system; (2) chorionic villus sampling
CVVH — continuous veno-venous haemofiltration
CVVHD — continuous veno-venous haemodialfiltration
Cx — cervix
CXR — chest X-ray

cm ― センチメートル

CML ― 慢性骨髄性白血病

CMV ― サイトメガロウイルス

CNS ― (1) 中枢神経系；(2) 臨床専門看護師

C/O ― 〜を訴える

COPD ― 慢性閉塞性肺疾患

COSHH ― 有害物質管理規則

CPA ― ケア・プログラム・アプローチ〔地域において精神疾患患者の日常的なケアを強化することにより，病床での負担削減を目的とする〕

CPAP ― 持続的気道内陽圧（呼吸）〔人口呼吸の方法〕

CPD ― 専門職継続開発訓練〔制度〕

CPN ― 地域精神医学専門看護師

CPR ― 心肺蘇生法

CRF ― 慢性腎不全

CSCI ― 社会的ケア検査委員会〔NHS の社会的ケアサービスの適切さを検査する独立機関〕

CSF ― (1) 脳脊髄液；(2) コロニー刺激因子

CSI ― 介護者負担指標

CSSD ― 中央材料滅菌室，中央滅菌供給部

CSU ― カテーテルによる採尿

CT ― (1) コンピュータ断層撮影法；(2) 冠動脈血栓（症）

CTG ― 胎児心拍陣痛計，分娩監視装置

CV ― (1) 心血管系の；(2) 履歴書

CVA ― 脳血管障害

CVP ― 中心静脈圧

CVS ― (1) 心血管系；(2) 絨毛生検

CVVH ― 持続的静脈・静脈血液濾過

CVVHD ― 持続的静脈・静脈血液濾過透析

Cx ― 頚（くび），子宮頸管

CXR ― 胸部 X 線写真

D

DADL — Domestic Activities of Daily Living
D&C — dilatation and curettage
DC — direct current
DDH — developmental dysplasia of the hip
DIC — disseminated intravascular coagulation
DipEd — Diploma in Education
DipHE — Diploma in Higher Education
DipN — Diploma in Nursing
DipNEd — Diploma in Nursing Education
DKA — diabetic ketoacidosis
DM — diabetes mellitus
DN — district nurse
DNA — (1) deoxyribonucleic acid; (2) did not attend
DOA — dead on arrival
DOB — date of birth
DoH — Department of Health
DPhil — Doctor of Philosophy
DRS — Delusions Rating Scale
DRV — dietary reference value
DSH — deliberate self-harm
DT — delirium tremens
DTPer — diphtheria, tetanus and pertussis vaccine
DU — duodenal ulcer
DVT — deep venous thrombosis
D&V — diarrhoea and vomiting
DXR — deep X-ray radiation
DXT — deep X-ray therapy

D

DADL ― 家での日常生活動作

D&C ― 頚管拡張子宮内膜搔爬術

DC ― 直流

DDH ― 発達性股関節脱臼，発育的股関節形成異常

DIC ― 播種性血管内凝固症候群

DipEd ― 教育学学位

DipHE ― 高等教育学位

DipN ― 看護学学位

DipNEd ― 看護教育学学位

DKA ― 糖尿病性ケトアシドーシス

DM ― 糖尿病

DN ― 地区看護師〔日本における訪問看護師のような活動をしている〕

DNA ― (1) デオキシリボ核酸；(2) 予約があるのに現れなかった患者

DOA ― 来院時既死亡〔brought in dead; BID「入院時死亡」と同意〕

DOB ― 生年月日

DoH ― 〔英国〕保険医療省

DPhil ― 〔英国の〕博士号〔PhD と略されることもある〕

DRS ― 妄想評価尺度

DRV ― 食事摂取基準

DSH ―「故意に自分の健康を害する」症候群，故意の自傷行為

DT ― 振戦せん妄

DTPer ― ジフテリア・破傷風・百日咳3種混合ワクチン

DU ― 十二指腸潰瘍

DVT ― 深部静脈血栓〔症〕

D&V ― 下痢と嘔吐

DXR ― X線深部照射

DXT ― X線深部療法

E

EAR — estimated average requirement
EBM — expressed breast milk
EBP — evidence-based practice
EBS — emergency bed service
EBV — Epstein-Barr virus
ECF — extracellular fluid
ECG — electrocardiogram
ECI — Experience of Caregiving Inventory
ECMO — extracorporeal membrane oxygenator
ECT — electroconvulsive therapy
EDC — expected date of confinement
EDD — expected date of delivery
EEG — electroencephalogram
EFAs — essential fatty acids
ELISA — enzyme-linked immunosorbent assay
EMD — electromechanical dissociation
EMG — electromyography
EMLA — eutectic mixture of local anaesthetics
EMU — early morning specimen of urine
ENT — ears, nose and throat
EOG — electro-oculogram
ERCP — endoscopic retrograde cholangiopancreatography
ERG — electroretinogram
ERPC — evacuation of retained products of conception
ERV — expiratory reserve volume
ESR — erythrocyte sedimentation rate
ESRD — end-stage renal disease
ESS — Early Signs Scale

E

EAR ― 推定平均必要量

EBM ― 搾った母乳

EBP ― 科学的根拠に基づく実践

EBS ― 緊急病床サービス〔英国国内の，受け入れ可能な集中治療病床の探索を調整する〕

EBV ― エプスタイン・バー・ウイルス〔EB ウイルスとも言う〕

ECF ― 細胞外液

ECG ― 心電図

ECI ― 介護者経験評価尺度

ECMO ― 体外式膜型人工肺

ECT ― 電気ショック療法

EDC ― 分娩予定日

EDD ― 分娩予定日

EEG ― 脳波図

EFAs ― 必須脂肪酸

ELISA ― 酵素結合免疫吸着測定法

EMD ― 電気収縮解離

EMG ― 筋電図検査

EMLA ― 局所麻酔剤共融混合物

EMU ― 早朝尿検体

ENT ― 耳，鼻，喉

EOG ― 電気眼球図

ERCP ― 内視鏡的逆行性胆管膵管造影〔法〕

ERG ― 網膜電位図

ERPC ― 残留受胎産物の除去

ERV ― 呼気予備量

ESR ― 赤血球沈降速度

ESRD ― 末期腎不全

ESS ― 〔病気の〕早期兆候尺度

ESWL — extracorporeal shock wave lithotripsy
ET — (1) embryo transfer; (2) endotracheal
EUA — examination under anaesthesia

F

F — (1) Fahrenheit (temperature scale); (2) female
FAS — fetal alcohol syndrome
FB — foreign body
FBC — full blood count
FBS — fasting blood sugar
FETC — Further Education Teaching Certificate
FEV — forced expiratory volume
FFP — fresh frozen plasma
FH — (1) family history; (2) fetal heart
FHH — fetal heart heard
FHNH — fetal heart not heard
FMF — fetal movement felt
FPC — Family Planning Clinic
FPCert — Family Planning Certificate
FRC — functional residual capacity
FRCN — Fellow of the Royal College of Nursing
FSH — follicle stimulating hormone
FTND — full-term normal delivery
FVC — forced vital capacity

G

g — gram
GA — general anaesthetic

ESWL ― 体外衝撃波結石破砕術
ET ― (1) 胚移植 (2) 気管内
EUA ― 麻酔下での検査

F

F ― (1) 華氏 (温度目盛); (2) 女性
FAS ― 胎児性アルコール症候群〔アルコール依存症の母親から生まれた新生児に見られることがある〕
FB ― 異物
FBC ― 全血球計算〔CBC ― complete blood count とも言う〕
FBS ― 空腹時血糖
FETC ― 継続教育教授資格〔義務教育後の大学以外での場で教育を教える資格〕
FEV ― 努力肺活量〔FVC と同じ〕
FFP ― 新鮮凍結血漿
FH ― (1) 家族歴; (2) 胎児心臓
FHH ― 胎児の心音が聴かれる
FHNH ― 胎児の心音が聴かれない
FMF ― 胎動が感じられる
FPC ― ファミリー・プラン診療所〔避妊, 妊娠, 性感染症などについての助言指導, 検査などを行う〕
FPCert ― ファミリー・プラン履修証明書〔避妊, 妊娠, 性感染症などに関する専門知識を習得している医師・看護師などに与えられる〕
FRC ― 機能的残気量
FRCN ― 王立看護協会の会員〔王立看護協会は看護師の生涯学習を推進しており, 会員は図書館や情報提供サービスなどを受けることができる〕
FSH ― 卵胞刺激ホルモン
FTND ― 満期正常分娩
FVC ― 努力肺活量〔FEV と同じ〕

G

g ― グラム
GA ― 全身麻酔

GC — gonococcus
GCS — Glasgow Coma Scale
GFR — glomerular filtration rate
GGT — γ-glutamyl transferase
GH — growth hormone
GHQ — General Health Questionnaire
GI — gastrointestinal
GIFT — gamete intrafallopian transfer
GIT — gastrointestinal tract
GOR — gastro-oesophageal reflux
GP — general practitioner
GSL — General Sales List (medicines)
GTN — glycelyl trinitrate
GTT — glucose tolerance test
GU — (1) gastric ulcer; (2) genitourinary
GUM — genitourinary medicine
GUS — genitourinary system
GVHD — graft versus host disease
Gyn — gynaecology

H

HAI — hospital-acquired infection
HAV — hepatitis A virus
HAVS — hand-arm vibration syndrome
Hb — haemoglobin
HBIG — hepatitis B immunoglobulin
HBV — hepatitis B virus
HC — head circumference
HCA — healthcare assistant

GC ― 淋菌

GCS ― グラスゴー・コーマ・スケール

GFR ― 糸球体濾過量

GGT ― ガンマグルタミルトランスフェラーゼ

GH ― 成長ホルモン

GHQ ― GHQ 精神健康調査票

GI ― 胃腸

GIFT ― 配偶子卵管内移植

GIT ― 消化管

GOR ― 胃食道逆流

GP ― 一般開業医〔英国では発病した際には「かかりつけ医」として，まず登録してある GP の診察を受ける〕

GSL ― 自由販売品（薬品）

GTN ― ニトログリセリン

GTT ― ブドウ糖負荷試験

GU ― (1) 胃潰瘍；(2) 腎尿路生殖器の，泌尿生殖器の，尿路性器の

GUM ― 腎尿路生殖器科学，泌尿生殖器科学，尿路性器科学

GUS ― 腎尿路生殖器系，泌尿生殖器系，尿路性器系

GVHD ― 移植片対宿主病

Gyn ― 婦人科〔学〕

H

HAI ― 院内感染，病院感染

HAV ― A 型肝炎ウイルス

HAVS ― 手腕振動症候群

Hb ― ヘモグロビン，血色素

HBIG ― B 型肝炎免疫グロブリン

HBV ― B 型肝炎ウイルス

HC ― 頭囲

HCA ― 保健ケア・アシスタント〔1990 年より英国の NHS の医療従事者として新しく生まれた職種である。専門家の補助的存在として病院やコミュニティで活動している〕

HCG (hCG) — human chorionic gonadotrophin
HCV — hepatitis C virus
HDL — high-density lipoprotein
HDSU — Hospital Disinfection and Sterilisation Unit
HDU — High Dependency Unit
HDV — hepatitis D virus
HEV — hepatitis E virus
HFEA — Human Fertilisation and Embryology Authority
HHNK — hyperglycaemic hyperosmolar non-ketotic
HI — head injury
Hib vaccine — Haemophilus influenzae type B vaccine
HImP — Health Improvement Programme
HIV — human immunodeficiency virus
HNPU — has not passed urine
HoNOS — Health of the Nation Outcome Scale
HPA — Health Protection Agency
HPV — human papilloma virus
HR — heart rate
HRS — Hallucinations Rating Scale
HRT — hormone-replacement therapy
HSV — herpes simplex virus
Ht — height
HUS — haemolytic uraemic syndrome
HV — Health Visitor
HVCert — Health Visitor's Certificate
HVT — Health Visitor Teacher

HCG (hCG) ― ヒト絨毛性ゴナドトロピン，ヒト絨毛性性腺刺激ホルモン
HCV ― C型肝炎ウイルス
HDL ― 高密度リポタンパク質
HDSU ― 消毒・滅菌ユニット
HDU ― 重症ケアユニット〔集中医療質と一般病棟の間に位置する〕
HDV ― D型肝炎ウイルス
HEV ― E型肝炎ウイルス
HFEA ― ヒト受精・胚機構
HHNK ― 非ケトン性高浸透圧性高血糖の
HI ― 頭部外傷，頭部損傷
Hib vaccine ― インフルエンザ菌b型ワクチン
HImP ― 健康改善プログラム〔医療と福祉が連携して各地域の健康と福祉の改善を目指す〕
HIV ― ヒト免疫不全ウイルス
HNPU ― 排尿なし
HoNOS ― 国家健康成果尺度〔精神健康の障害の度数を測る〕
HPA ― 健康保護局
HPV ― ヒトパピローマウイルス，ヒト乳頭腫ウイルス
HR ― 心拍数
HRS ― 幻覚評価尺度
HRT ― ホルモン補充療法
HSV ― 単純ヘルペスウイルス
Ht ― 身長
HUS ― 溶血性尿毒症症候群
HV ― 巡回保健師〔コミュニティで保健活動すべくトレーニングを積んだ看護師や助産師のこと〕
HVCert ― 訪問保健師資格
HVT ― 教授資格のある訪問保健師〔保健師を目指す学生を教える〕

I

IABP — intra-aortic balloon pump
IADL — Instrumental Activities of Daily Living
IBD — intflammatory bowel disease
IBS — irritable bowel syndrome
IC — inspiratory capacity
ICD — International Classification of Disease
ICE — ice, compress and elevate
ICF — intracellular fluid
ICN — (1) Infection Control Nurse; (2) International Council of Nurses
ICP — intracranial pressure
ICSH — interstitial cell stimulating hormone
ICU — Intensive Care Unit
ID — infectious disease
IDDM — insulin-dependent diabetes mellitus
IE — infective endocarditis
IGT — impaired glucose tolerance
IHD — ischaemic heart disease
IM — (1) infectious mononucleosis; (2) intramuscular
IMV — intermittent mandatory ventilation
INR — (1) Index of Nursing Research; (2) international normalised ratio
IOP — intraocular pressure
IPD — intermittent peritoneal dialysis
IPP — intermittent positive pressure
IPPV — intermittent positive pressure ventilation
IQ — intelligence quotient
IRV — inspiratory reserve volume
IS — Insight Scale

I

IABP ― 動脈内バルーンポンプ

IADL ― 手段的日常生活動作〔食事の準備，金銭管理，買い物などの具体的な生活手段の遂行能力のこと〕

IBD ― 炎症性腸疾患

IBS ― 過敏性腸症候群

IC ― 最大吸気量

ICD ― 国際疾病分類

ICE ― 氷で冷却し，圧迫して，挙上する〔出血を伴わない急性外傷時の応急処置として知られている〕

ICF ― 細胞内液

ICN ―（1）感染管理認定看護師；（2）国際看護師協会

ICP ― 頭蓋内圧

ICSH ― 間質細胞刺激ホルモン〔LHと同一のホルモン〕

ICU ― 集中治療室

ID ― 感染症

IDDM ― インスリン依存性糖尿病

IE ― 感染性心内膜炎

IGT ― 耐糖能障害

IHD ― 虚血性心疾患

IM ―（1）伝染性単核症（2）筋肉内

IMV ― 間欠的強制呼吸

INR ―（1）看護研究インデックス（2）国際標準化率

IOL ― 眼内レンズ

IOP ― 眼内圧

IPD ― 間欠的腹膜透析

IPP ― 間欠的陽圧呼吸

IPPV ― 間欠的陽圧換気法

IQ ― 知能指数

IRV ― 予備呼気量

IS ― 病識尺度

IT — information technology
ITU — Intensive Therapy Unit
IU — international unit
IUD — intrauterine (contraceptive) device
IUI — intrauterine insemination
IV — intravenous
IVC — inferior vena cava
IVF — in vitro fertilisation
IVI — intravenous infusion
IVU — intravenous urogram

J

JCA — juvenile chronic arthritis
JVP — jugular venous pressure

K

KASI — Knowledge about Schizophrenia Interview
KS — Kaposi's sarcoma
KUB — kidney, ureter and bladder

L

L, l — litre
LA — (1) left atrium; (2) local anaesthetic; (3) local authority
lb — pound (of weight)
LBP — low back pain
LDH — lactate dehydrogenase
LDL — low-density lipoprotein
LDQ — Leeds Dependence Questionnaire
LFTs — liver function tests
LH — luteinising hormone
LIF — left iliac fossa

IT ― 情報技術

ITU ― 集中治療部

IU ― 国際単位

IUD ― 子宮内避妊具

IUI ― 子宮内人工授精

IV ― 静脈内

IVC ― 下大静脈

IVF ― 体外受精

IVI ― 点滴静注

IVU ― 静脈性尿路造影

J

JCA ― 若年性関節リウマチ

JVP ― 頚静脈圧

K

KASI ― 統合失調症知識面接

KS ― カポジ肉腫

KUB ― 腎・尿管・膀胱〔単純 X 線撮影〕

L

L, l ― リットル

LA ―（1）左心房；（2）局所麻酔；（3）地方自治体

lb ― ポンド（重量の単位：454g に相当）

LBP ― 腰痛

LDH ― 乳酸デヒドロゲナーゼ

LDL ― 低密度リポタンパク質

LDQ ― リーズ依存性調査票

LFTs ― 肝機能検査

LH ― 黄体形成ホルモン

LIF ― 左腸骨窩

LMN — lower motor neuron
LMP — last menstrual period
LOC — level of consciousness
LP — lumbar puncture
LRNI — lower reference nutrient intake
LRTI — lower respiratory tract infection
LSCS — lower segment Caesarean section
LTM — long-term memory
LUNSERS — Liverpool University Neuroleptic Side Effect Rating Scale
LV — left ventricle
LVAD — left ventricular assist device
LVF — left ventricular failure
LVH — left ventricular hypertrophy

M

M — male
MA — Master of Arts
MAC — mid-arm circumference
mane — in the morning (of drugs); tomorrow
MAO — monoamine oxidase inhibitor
MBC — maximal breathing capacity
MCA — Medicines Control Agency (now merged with Medical Devices Agency)
MCH — mean cell haemoglobin
MCHC — mean cell haemoglobin concentration
MCL — mid-clavicular line
MCV — mean cell volume
MDA — Medical Devices Agency (now merged with Medicines Control Agency)
MDR-TB — multidrug resistant tuberculosis

LMN ― 下位運動ニューロン

LMP ― 最終月経，最終月経期

LOC ― 意識レベル

LP ― 腰椎穿刺

LRNI ― 最低基準栄養所要量

LRTI ― 下気道感染〔症〕

LSCS ― 子宮下部帝王切開

LTM ― 長期記憶

LUNSERS ― リバプール大学神経遮断副作用評価尺度

LV ― 左心室

LVAD ― 左室補助装置

LVF ― 左室不全

LVH ― 左室肥大

M

M ― 男性

MA ― 文学修士

MAC ― 上腕周囲長

mane ― 朝に；翌日に〔薬剤投与におけるラテン語表現〕

MAO ― モノアミンオキシダーゼン阻害薬

MBC ― 分時最大呼吸量，分時最大換気量

MCA ― 〔英国〕医薬品管理局（現在は医療用品規制局と統合）

MCH ― 赤血球ヘモグロビンを意味する

MCHC ― 赤血球ヘモグロビン濃度を意味する

MCL ― 鎖骨中央線

MCV ― 平均赤血球容積

MDA ― 〔英国〕医療用品規制局（現在は医薬品管理局と統合）

MDR-TB ― 多剤耐性結核

ME — myalgic encephalomyelitis
MEd — Master of Education
M/F; M/W/S/D — male/female; married/widowed/single/divorced
MHRA — Medicines and Healthcare products Regulatory Agency (formed from the MCA and MDA)
MI — (1) mitral incompetence or insufficiency; (2) myocardial infarction
mmHg — millimetres of mercury
mmol — millimole
MMR — measles mumps and rubella (as in vaccine)
MMV — mandatory minute volume
MODS — multiple organ dysfunction syndrome
MODY — maturity onset diabetes of the young
MPhil — Master of Philosophy
MRI — magnetic resonance imaging
MRSA — methicillin-resistant Staphylococcus aureus
MS — (1) mitral stenosis; (2) multiple sclerosis; (3) musculoskeletal
MSc — Master of Science
MSH — melanocytestimulating hormone
MSP — Munchausen syndrome by proxy
MSU — mid-stream urine
MSW — medical social worker
MT — midwifery teacher
MTD — Midwife Teachers' Diploma
MWO — mental welfare officer

N

NAD — no abnormality detected
NAI — non-accidental injury
NAS — no added salt

ME ― 筋痛性脳脊髄炎

MEd ― 教育学修士

M/F; M/W /S/D ― 男性 / 女性；既婚 / 死別 / 独身 / 離婚

MHRA ―〔英国〕医薬品・医療製品規制庁（医薬品管理局と医療品規制局から成る）

MI ―（1）僧帽弁閉鎖不全症または機能不全（2）心筋梗塞

mmHg ― ミリメートル水銀柱

mmol ― ミリモル

MMR ― 麻疹・おたふく風邪・風疹（ワクチンで）

MMV ― 強制分時換気量

MODS ― 多臓器障害

MODY ― 若年発症成人型糖尿病

MPhil ― 研究重視の修士号

MRI ― 磁気共鳴画像診断

MRSA ― メチシリン耐性黄色ブドウ球菌

MS ―（1）僧帽弁狭窄（2）多発性硬化症（3）筋骨格

MSc ― 理学修士

MSH ― メラニン細胞刺激ホルモン

MSP ― 代理ミュンヒハウゼン症候群

MSU ― 中間尿

MSW ― 医療ソーシャルワーカー

MT ― 教授資格のある助産師〔大学，病院，地域などで助産学を教える〕

MTD ― 助産師教授学位

MWO ― 精神保健福祉職員

N

NAD ― 検査異常なし

NAI ― 非偶発的損傷

NAS ― 塩分無添加

NBI — no bone injury
NBM — nil (nothing) by mouth
NCVQ — National Council for Vocational Qualifications
ND — normal delivery
NFA — (1) no fixed abode; (2) no further action
NG — nasogastric
NHL — non-Hodgkin's lymphoma
NHS — National Health Service
NICE — National Institute for Clinical Excellence
NICU — Neonatal Intensive Care Unit
NIDDM — non-insulindependent diabetes mellitus
NIPPV — non-invasive positive pressure ventilation
NMC — Nursing and Midwifery Council
NMR — nuclear magnetic resonance
nocte — in the evening (of drugs)
NPF — Nurse Prescribers' Formulary
NPU — not passed urine
NRDS — neonatal respiratory distress syndrome
NREM — non-rapid eye movement (sleep)
NSAIDs — non-steroidal antiintflammatory drugs
NSFs — National Service Frameworks
NSP — non-starch polysaccharides
NSU — non-specific urethritis
NT — nurse teacher
N&V — nausea and vomiting
NVQ — National Vocational Qualification

NBI ― 骨に損傷なし

NBM ― 絶食

NCVQ ― 全国職業資格委員会

ND ― 正常分娩

NFA ― (1) 住所不定 (2) これ以上の処置必要なし

NG ― 経鼻的胃

NHL ― 非ホジキンリンパ腫

NHS ―〔英国の〕国民健康保険〔原則的に無料で医療サービスが受けられるが，財政難や受診までの長い待ち時間などが問題となっている〕

NICE ― 国立臨床評価機構

NICU ― 新生児集中治療室

NIDDM ― インスリン非依存性糖尿病

NIPPV ― 非侵襲的陽圧的換気，非侵襲的陽圧的人工呼吸

NMC ― 看護師助産師会

NMR ― 核磁気共鳴分析

nocte ― 夜に，寝る前に（薬の服用）〔ラテン語 ― 薬の服用を「夜に」行うよう指示の際に使われることがある〕

NPF ― 処方看護師のための処方書〔英国では処方資格を有する看護師は限定的な処方が可能〕

NPU ― 排尿なし

NRDS ― 新生児呼吸促迫症候群

NREM ― ノンレム睡眠

NSAIDs ― 非ステロイド性抗炎症薬

NSFs ―〔英国〕医療サービス・フレームワーク〔医療サービスの向上を目指した戦略的目標〕

NSP ― 非澱粉多糖体

NSU ― 非特異性尿道炎

NT ― 養護教諭

N&V ― 悪心嘔吐

NVQ ― 全国職業検定資格

O

OA — osteoarthritis
OBS — organic brain syndrome
OCD — obsessive-compulsive disorder
o.d. — omni die (Latin — sometimes used in prescriptions), daily
OD — overdose
ODP — operating department practitioner
O/E, OE — on examination
OGD — oesophagogastroduodenoscopy
OHNC — Occupational Health Nursing Certificate
o.m. — omni mane (Latin — sometimes used in prescriptions), in the morning
o.n. — omni nocte (Latin — sometimes used in prescriptions), at night
ONC — Orthopaedic Nurses' Certificate
OND — Ophthalmic Nursing Diploma
OPCS — Office of Population Censuses and Surveys
OPD — Outpatients Department
ORT — oral rehydration therapy
OT — occupational therapist (therapy)
OTC — over the counter (drugs bought without a prescription)
OU — Open University

P

P — pulse
PAC — premature atrial contraction
PADL — Personal Activities of Daily Living
PAFC — pulmonary artery flotation catheter
PALS — paediatric advanced life support
PANSS — Positive and Negative Syndrome Scale
Pap — Papanicolaou smear test

O

OA ― 骨関節症
OBS ― 器質性脳症候群
OCD ― 強迫性障害
o.d. ― 毎日（ラテン語 ― 処方箋に使われることがある）
OD ―〔薬物の〕過量，過剰投与，過剰服用
ODP ― 手術部専門職〔患者のケア，手術器具の準備，術中の外科医の第一アシスタントなどを行う〕
O/E, OE ― 検査の上で
OGD ― 食道胃十二指腸鏡検査
OHNC ― 産業保険看護師認定資格
o.m. ― 午前中に（ラテン語 ― 処方箋でときどき使用される）
o.n. ― 夜間に（ラテン語 ― 処方箋でときどき使用される）
ONC ― 整形外科看護師資格
OND ― 眼科看護学位
OPCS ―〔英国の〕国勢調査局
OPD ― 外来診療部
ORT ― 経口補水塩療法
OT ― 作業療法士（作業療法）
OTC ― 店頭販売〔薬〕（処方箋なしで購入する薬）
OU ― 放送大学

P

P ― 脈
PAC ― 心房性期外収縮
PADL ― 個人的日常生活動作
PAFC ― 肺動脈浮遊カテーテル，スワン・ガンツカテーテル
PALS ― 小児二次救命処置
PANSS ― 陽性・陰性症状評価尺度
Pap ― パパニコロー・スミア試験

PAT — paroxysmal atrial tachycardia
PAWP — pulmonary artery wedge pressure
PBD — peak bone density
PBM — peak bone mass
p.c. — post cibum (Latin — sometimes used in prescriptions), after food
PCAG — primary closed-angle glaucoma
PCA(S) — patient-controlled analgesia (system)
PCEA — patient-controlled epidural analgesia
PCM — protein-calorie malnutrition
PCP — Pneumocystis carinii pneumonia
PCT — Primary Care Trust
PCV — packed cell volume
PCWP — pulmonary capillary wedge pressure
PD — peritoneal dialysis
PDA — patent ductus arteriosus
PDP — personal development plan
PE — pulmonary embolus
PEEP — positive endexpiratory pressure
PEFR — peak expiratory flow rate
PEG — percutaneous endoscopic gastrostomy
PEM — protein-energy malnutrition
PET — (1) positron emission tomography; (2) preeclamptic toxaemia
PFI — private finance initiative
PFR — peak flow rate
PGL — persistent generalised lymphadenopathy
pH — hydrogen ion concentration
PHCT — Primary Health Care Team
PhD — Doctor of Philosophy

PAT — 発作性心房性頻拍〔症〕

PAWP — 肺動脈楔入圧

PBD — 最大骨密度

PBM — 最大骨量

p.c. — 食後（ラテン語 — ときどき処方箋で使われる）

PCAG — 原発閉塞隅角緑内障

PCA(S) — 自己調節鎮痛，自己疼痛管理，患者管理無痛

PCEA — 自己調節硬膜外鎮痛

PCM — タンパク質・エネルギー栄養失調症

PCP — カリニ肺炎

PCT — プライマリー・ケア・トラスト〔適正な地域医療サービスの監視，資金などの管理を行う公益法人〕

PCV — ヘマトクリット値

PCWP — 肺毛細血管楔入圧

PD — 腹膜透析

PDA — 動脈管開存〔症〕

PDP — 個人開発計画

PE — 肺塞栓

PEEP — 呼気終末陽圧

PEFR — 最大呼気流量

PEG — 胃瘻，経皮内視鏡的胃瘻造設術

PEM — タンパク質エネルギー栄養障害

PET — (1) ポジトロン放射形断層撮影 (2) 子癇前症性中毒症

PFI — 民間資金活用事業〔民間の資金・スキルなどを利用して公共施設などを整備・運用する手法〕

PFR — 最大流量

PGL — 持続性全身性リンパ節腫脹

pH — 水素イオン濃度

PHCT — プライマリー・ヘルス・ケア・チーム〔地域の医療専門職で構成され，初期治療を提供する〕

PhD — 博士号

PHLS — Public Health Laboratory Service
PICC — peripherally inserted central catheter
PICU — Paediatric Intensive Care Unit
PID — (1) pelvic inflammatory disease; (2) prolapsed intervertebral disc
PKU — phenylketonuria
PL — perception of light
PM — postmortem
PMB — postmenopausal bleeding
PMH — past medical history
PMS — premenstrual syndrome
PMT — premenstrual tension
PN — postnatal
PND — paroxysmal nocturnal dyspnoea
POAG — primaly open-angle glaucoma
POM — prescription only medicine
PONV — postoperative nausea and vomiting
POP — plaster of Paris
PPD — (1) progressive perceptive deafness; (2) purified protein derivative
PPH — post-partum haemorrhage
PPS — plasma protein solution
PPV — positive pressure ventilation
PR — per rectum
PREP — post-registration education and practice
PRL — prolactin
p.r.n. — pro re nata (Latin — sometimes used in prescriptions), when required
PSA — prostate-specific antigen

PHLS ― 公衆衛生検査サービス
PICC ― 末梢穿刺中心静脈カテーテル
PICU ― 小児集中医療室
PID ― (1) 骨盤内炎症性疾患 (2) 椎間板ヘルニア
PKU ― フェニルケトン尿症
PL ― 光覚
PM ― 〔副詞として〕死後に,〔名詞として〕検死
PMB ― 閉経後出血
PMH ― 既往歴
PMS ― 月経前症候群
PMT ― 月経前緊張
PN ― 生後,出産後
PND ― 発作性夜間呼吸困難
POAG ― 原発性開放隅角緑内障
POM ― 処方箋薬
PONV ― 術後悪心嘔吐
POP ― ギプス
PPD ― (1) 進行性感音難聴 (2) 精製ツベルクリン
PPH ― 分娩後出血
PPS ― 血漿タンパク質溶液
PPV ― 陽圧換気
PR ― 経直腸的に
PREP ― 看護師の生涯教育と実践制度〔看護師が登録後も継続して学び,高い水準の能力を維持するための制度〕
PRL ― プロラクチン
p.r.n. ― 必要に応じて(ラテン語 ― ときどき処方箋で使われる)
PSA ― 前立腺特異抗原

PSCT — Pain and Symptom Control Team
PSV — pressure support ventilation
PT — (1) physiotherapist; (2) prothrombin
PTA — prior to admission
PTC — percutaneous transhepatic cholangiography
PTCA — percutaneous transluminal coronary angioplasty
PTH — parathyroid hormone
PTSD — post-traumatic stress disorder
PTT — partial thromboplastin time
PU — passed urine
PUFA — polyunsaturated fatty acid
PUO — pyrexia of unknown origin
PV — per vagina
PVD — peripheral vascular disease
PVS — persistent vegetative state
PVT — paroxysmal ventricular tachycardia

Q

QALY — quality-adjusted lifeyear
q.d.s. — quater die sumendus (Latin — sometimes used in prescriptions), four times a day
q.i.d. — quater in die (Latin), four times a day
QIDN — Queen's Institute of District Nursing
q.q.h. — quarta quaque hora (Latin), every 4 hours

R

R — respiration
RA — (1) rheumatoid arthritis; (2) right atrium
RAI — Relatives' Assessment Interview
RAISSE — Relatives' Assessment Interview for Schizophrenia in a

PSCT ― 疼痛・症状対策チーム

PSV ― 圧支持換気

PT ―（1）理学療法士（2）プロトロンビン

PTA ― 入院前に

PTC ― 経皮経肝〔的〕胆管造影〔撮影〕〔法〕

PTCA ― 経皮的冠〔状〕〔動脈〕形成〔術〕

PTH ― 上皮小体ホルモン，副甲状腺ホルモン

PTSD ― 心的外傷後ストレス障害

PTT ― 部分トロンボプラスチン時間

PU ― 排尿あり

PUFA ― 多価不飽和脂肪酸

PUO ― 原因不明熱

PV ― 腟を通して

PVD ― 末梢血管疾患

PVS ― 遷延性意識障害

PVT ― 発作性心室性頻拍

Q

QALY ― 質調整生存年

q.d.s. ― 1日4回（ラテン語 ― ときどき処方箋で使われる）

q.i.d. ― 1日4回（ラテン語）

QIDN ― 地域看護師協会〔現在は Queen's Nursing Institute「看護師協会」〕

q.q.h. ― 4時間ごとに（ラテン語）

R

R ― 呼吸

RA ―（1）関節リウマチ（2）右心房

RAI ― 親族評価面接〔精神疾患患者の親族による介入の影響を測る〕

RAISSE ― 安定した環境における統合失調症のための親族評価面接〔RAIの1つ〕

Secure Environment

RBC — (1) red blood cell; (2) red blood cell count
RBS — random blood sugar
RCC — red cell concentrate
RCM — Royal College of Midwives
RCN — Royal College of Nursing and National Council of Nurses of the UK
RCNT — Registered Clinical Nurse Teacher
RCT — randomised controlled trial
RDA — recommended daily allowance
REM — rapid eye movement (sleep)
RG — remedial gymnast
RGN — Registered General Nurse
Rh — rhesus factor
RHD — rheumatic heart disease
RHV — Registered Health Visitor
RICE — rest, ice, compress, elevation
RIF — right iliac fossa
rINN — recommended international non-proprietary name
RIP — raised intracranial pressure
RM — Registered Midwife
RMN — Registered Mental Nurse
RN — Registered Nurse
RNA — ribonucleic acid
RNI — reference nutrient intake
RNIB — Royal National Institute for the Blind
RNID — Royal National Institute for the Deaf
RNMH — Registered Nurse for the Mentally Handicapped
RNT — Registered Nurse Tutor
RO — reality orientation

RBC ― (1) 赤血球 (2) 赤血球数
RBS ― 任意血糖
RCC ― 赤血球濃厚液
RCM ― 英国王立助産師大学
RCN ― 英国王立看護大学
RCNT ― 正臨床看護師教官
RCT ― 無作為対照試験
RDA ― 1日あたりの推奨摂取量
REM ― 急速眼球運動，レム睡眠
RG ― 治療体操師
RGN ― 正看護師
Rh ― Rh因子
RHD ― リウマチ性心疾患
RHV ― 正巡回保健師
RICE ― 安静にし，氷で冷却し，圧迫して，挙上する
RIF ― 右腸骨窩
rINN ― 推奨国際一般名
RIP ― 頭蓋内圧亢進
RM ― 正助産師
RMN ― 精神科専門看護師
RN ― 正看護師
RNA ― リボ核酸
RNI ― 推奨栄養摂取量
RNIB ― 王立視覚障害者協会
RNID ― 王立聴覚障害者協会
RNMH ― 精神障害専門正看護師
RNT ― 正看護師指導教官
RO ― 現実見当識訓練

ROM — range of movement (exercises)
ROS — removal of sutures
RS — respiratory system
RSCN — Registered Sick Children's Nurse
RSI — repetitive strain injury
RSV — respiratory syncytial virus
RTA — (1) renal tubular acidosis; (2) road traffic accident
RTI — respiratory tract infection
RV — (1) residual volume; (2) right ventricle
RVF — right ventricular failure

S

SAD — seasonal affective disorder
SAH – subarachnoidal haemorrhage
SAI — sexually acquired infection
SANS — Schedule for Assessment of Negative Symptoms
SARS — severe acute respiratory syndrome
SC — subcutaneous
SCBU — Special Care Baby Unit
SCC — (1) spinal cord compression; (2) squamous cell carcinoma
SCD — sequential pneumatic compression device
SCM — State Certified Midwife
SDAT — senile dementia Alzheimer type
SDH — subdural haematoma
SERMs — selective (o)estrogen receptor modulators
SFS — Social Functioning Scale
SG — specific gravity
SGA — small for gestational age
SHHD — Scottish Home and Health Department
SHO — senior house officer

ROM ― 可動域（運動）

ROS ― 抜糸

RS ― 呼吸器系

RSCN ― 小児専門看護師

RSI ― 反復過多損傷

RSV ― RS ウイルス，呼吸系発疹ウイルス

RTA ―（1）尿細管性アシドーシス（2）道路交通事故

RTI ― 気道感染

RV ―（1）残気量（2）右心室

RVF ― 右心不全

S

SAD ― 季節的情動障害

SAH ― くも膜下出血

SAI ― 性行為感染症

SANS ― 陰性症状評価尺度〔統合失調症の陰性症状の診断指標〕

SARS ― 重症急性呼吸器症候群

SC ― 皮下の

SCBU ― 新生児特別治療室

SCC ―（1）脊髄圧迫（2）扁平細胞癌

SCD ― 間欠連続性空気圧縮装置

SCM ― 国家公認助産師

SDAT ― アルツハイマー型老年認知症

SDH ― 硬膜下血腫

SERMs ― 選択的エストロゲン受容体調節薬

SFS ― 社会機能評価尺度

SG ― 比重

SGA ― 胎内発育遅延，胎児発育遅延

SHHD ― スコットランド家庭健康省

SHO ― 医長

SI Units — Systéme International d'Unités
SIB — self-injurious behaviour
SIDS — sudden infant death syndrome
SIMV — synchronised intermittent mandatory ventilation
SLE — systemic lupus erythematosus
SLS — social and life skills
SLT — speech and language therapist (therapy)
SMR — (1) standardised mortality rate; (2) submucous resection
SNAP — Schizophrenia Nursing Assessment Protocol
SOB — short of breath
SPECT — single photon emission computed tomography
SPF — sun protection factor
SRN — State Registered Nurse
SSRIs — selective serotonin re-uptake inhibitors
stat. — statim (Latin — sometimes used in prescriptions), immediately
STD — sexually transmitted disease
STI — sexually transmitted infection
STM — short-term memory
STs — sanitary towels
SVC — superior vena cava
SVQs — Scottish Vocational Qualifications
SVT — supraventricular tachycardia
SWD - short-wave diathermy

T

T — temperature
T&A — tonsils and adenoids
TB — tuberculosis
TCA — tricyclic antidepressants
TCI — to come in

SI Units — 国際単位系
SIB — 自傷行為
SIDS — 乳幼児突然死症候群
SIMV — 同期型間欠的強制換気
SLE — 全身性エリテマトーデス
SLS — 社会的生活技能
SLT — 言語聴覚士（言語聴覚療法）
SMR — （1）標準化死亡率（2）窓形切除術
SNAP — 統合失調症看護評価プロトコール
SOB — 息切れ
SPECT — 単一光子放射形コンピュータ断層撮影法
SPF — 日焼け防止指数
SRN — 国家公認看護師
SSRIs — 選択的セロトニン再取り込み阻害薬
stat. — ただちに（ラテン語 — 処方箋でときどき使用される）
STD — 性感染症
STI — 性感染症
STM — 短期記憶
STs — 生理用ナプキン
SVC — 上大静脈
SVQs — スコットランド公認職業資格
SVT — 上室性頻拍症
SWD — 短波ジアテルミー

T

T — 温度，気温，体温，〔高い〕熱
T&A — 扁桃およびアデノイド
TB — 結核
TCA — 三環系抗うつ薬
TCI — 入院予定〔日〕

t.d.s. — ter die sumendus (Latin — sometimes used in prescriptions), three times a day

TEDs — thromboembolic deterrent (stockings)

TEN — toxic epidermal necrolysis

TENS — transcutaneous electrical nerve stimulation

TIA — transient ischaemic attack

t.i.d. — ter in die (Latin), three times a day

TIPSS — transjugular intrahepatic portasystemic stent shunting

TLC — total lung capacity

TLS — tumour lysis syndrome

TNF — tumour necrosis factor

TNM — tumour, node, metastasis

TOP — termination of pregnancy

TPN — total parenteral nutrition

TPR — temperature, pulse, respiration

TRIC — trachoma inclusion conjunctivitis

TSF — triceps skin-fold thickness

TSH — thyroid-stimulating hormone

TSS — toxic shock syndrome

TT — (1) tetanus toxoid; (2) thrombin clotting time; (3) tuberculin tested

TTA(O) — to take away (out)

TUR — transurethral resection

TURP — transurethral resection of the prostate gland

TURT — transurcthral resection of tumour

TV — (1) tidal volume; (2) Trichomonas vaginalis

U

U — unit

U&E — urea and electrolytes

t.d.s. ― 1日3回（ラテン語 ― 処方箋でときどき使用される）

TEDs ― 血栓塞栓症予防（ストッキング）

TEN ― 中毒性表皮壊死剥離症，中毒性表皮壊死融解

TENS ― 経皮的末梢神経電気刺激

TIA ― 一過性虚血発作

t.i.d. ― 1日3回（ラテン語）

TIPSS ― 経頚静脈性肝内門脈体循環短絡

TLC ― 総肺気量

TLS ― 腫瘍溶解症候群

TNF ― 腫瘍壊死因子

TNM ― TNM 分類，悪性腫瘍臨床国際分類

TOP ― 妊娠中絶

TPN ― 完全静脈栄養

TPR ― 体温，脈拍，呼吸

TRIC ― トラコーマ封入体結膜炎

TSF ― 上腕三頭筋皮下脂肪厚

TSH ― 甲状腺刺激ホルモン

TSS ― 毒素性ショック症候群

TT ― (1) 破傷風トキソイド；(2) トロンビン凝固時間；(3) ツベルクリン試験

TTA(O) ― 持ち帰り

TUR ― 経尿道的切除

TURP ― 経尿道的前立腺切除術

TURT ― 経尿道的腫瘍切除術

TV ― (1) b1 回呼吸気量；(2) 腟トリコモナス

U

U ― 単位

U&E ― 尿素と電解質

UG — urogenital
UGS — urogenital system
UGT — urogenital tract
UKCC — UK Central Council for Nursing, Midwifery and Health Visiting (replaced by Nursing and Midwifery Council)
UMN — upper motor neuron
URTI — upper respiratory tract infection
USS — ultrasound scan
UTI — urinary tract infection
UVA — ultraviolet A
UVB — ultraviolet B
UVL — ultraviolet light

V

VA — visual acuity
VAS — visual analogue scale
VBI — vertebrobasilar insufficiency
VC — vital capacity
VD — venereal disease (outdated term)
VE — vaginal examination
VF — ventricular fibrillation
VFM — value for money
VLDL — very-low-density lipoprotein
VRE — vancomycin-resistant enterococci
VRS — Verbal Rating Scale
VSD — ventricular septal defect
VT — ventricular tachycardia
VUR — vesicoureteric reflux
VV — varicose vein(s)
VZIG — varicella-zoster immunoglobulin

UG ― 腎尿路生殖器の

UGS ― 腎尿路生殖器系

UGT ― 腎尿路生殖器，尿路性器，尿生殖路

UKCC ― 英国看護助産訪問保健中央協議会（現在ではNMC「看護師助産師会」に代わっている）

UMN ― 上位運動ニューロン

URTI ― 上気道感染症

USS ― 超音波検査，超音波スキャン

UTI ― 尿路感染〔症〕

UVA ― 長波長紫外線

UVB ― 中波長紫外線

UVL ― 紫外線，紫外光

V

VA ― 視力

VAS ― 視覚的アナログ尺度，視覚的評価尺度

VBI ― 椎骨脳底動脈循環不全

VC ― 肺活量

VD ― 性病（現在では使われない旧式の用語）

VE ― 腟内診

VF ― 心室細動

VFM ― 金額に見合う価値，費用に値するだけの価値

VLDL ― 超低比重リポタンパク質

VRE ― バンコマイシン耐性腸球菌

VRS ― 言語評価尺度

VSD ― 心室中隔欠損〔症〕

VT ― 心室性頻拍，心室頻拍

VUR ― 膀胱尿管逆流

VV ― 静脈瘤

VZIG ― 水痘帯状疱疹免疫グロブリン

VZV — varicella-zoster virus

W

WBC — (1) white blood cell; (2) white blood cell count
WC — water closet (lavatory)
WHO — World Health Organisation
WPW — Wolff-Parkinson-White syndrome
Wt — weight

Z

ZIFT — zygote intrafallopian transfer
ZN — Ziehl-Neelsen (stain)

VZV ― 水痘帯状疱疹ウイルス

W

WBC ―（1）白血球；（2）白血球数
WC ― トイレ，水洗便所（洗面所，便所）
WHO ― 世界保健機関
WPW ― ウォルフ・パーキンソン・ホワイト症候群，WPW症候群
Wt ― 体重

Z

ZIFT ― 受精卵卵管内移植
ZN ― チール・ニールセン染色

IV Units of measurement

UNITS OF MEASUREMENT: INTERNATIONAL SYSTEM OF UNITS (SI), THE METRIC SYSTEM AND CONVERSIONS

In the UK we use the International System of Units (SI) or Système International d'Unités measurement system for scientific, medical and technical purposes, The SI units have replaced those of the Imperial System. For example, the kilogram is used for weight (or mass) instead of the pound, and the metre for length instead of yards, feet and inches. However, in everyday life you will still see a mix of units used in shops and hear people talk about pounds, and feet and inches. For example, they will ask for a pound of apples and describe someone being 5 foot 3 inches in height and 10 stone in weight.

The SI comprises seven base units, with several derived units. Each unit has its own symbol and is expressed as a decimal multiple or submultiple of the base unit by using the appropriate prefix (e.g. a millimetre is one-thousandth of a metre).

Base units

Quantity	Base unit and symbol
Length	metre (m)
Mass	kilogram (kg)
Time	second (s)
Amount of substance	mole (mol)
Electric current	ampere (A)
Thermodynamic temperature	kelvin (°K)
Luminous intensity	candela (cd)

Ⅳ　計量単位

計量単位：国際単位系 (SI)、メートル法と換算

英国では，国際単位系すなわち SI を科学的，医学的，技術的な用途において採用している。SI 法は英国度量法の代わりとして使われている。例えば，重さ（または質量）は，ポンドに代わりキログラムで，長さは，ヤード，フィート，インチに代わりメートルで表す。しかしながら，現在でもなお，日常生活では店先で両方の単位が混ざって使われているのを目にしたり，ポンドやフィート，インチが会話に出るのを耳にするだろう。1 ポンドのリンゴを買い求めたり，人を身長は 5 フィート 3 インチ，体重は 10 ストーンと描写するといった具合である。

　SI 単位は 7 つの基本単位といくつかの組立単位で構成されている。それぞれの単位には記号があり，適切な接頭辞を用い基本単位の十進法の倍数や約数で表される（例：1 ミリメートルは 1 メートルの 1000 分の 1）。

基本単位

量	基本単位と記号
長さ	メートル (m)
質量	キログラム (kg)
時間	秒 (s)
物質量	モル (mol)
電流	アンペア (A)
熱力学温度	ケルビン (°K)
光度	カンデラ (cd)

Derived units

Derived units for measuring different quantities are reached by multiplying or dividing two or more of the seven base units.

Quantity	Derived unit and symbol
Work. energy. quantity of heat	joule (J)
Pressure	pascal (Pa)
Force	newton (N)
Frequency	hertz (Hz)
Power	watt (W)
Electrical potential, electromotive force, potential difference	volt (v)
Absorbed dose of radiation	gray (Gy)
Radioactivity	becquerel (Bq)
Dose equivalent	sievert (Sv)

Factor, decimal multiples and submultiples of SI units

Multiplication factor	Prefix	Symbol
10^{12}	tera	T
10^{9}	giga	G
10^{6}	mega	M
10^{3}	kilo	k
10^{2}	hecto	h
10^{1}	deca	da
10^{-1}	deci	d
10^{-2}	centi	c
10^{-3}	milli	m

誘導（組立）単位

異なる量を測るための組立単位は，7つの基本単位を，2単位またはそれ以上の数の単位同士を掛けるか割るかによりできる。

量	組立単位と記号
仕事，エネルギー，熱量	ジュール (J)
圧力	パスカル (Pa)
力	ニュートン (N)
周波数，振動数	ヘルツ (Hz)
電力	ワット (W)
電位，起電力，電位差	ボルト (v)
放射線の吸収線量	グレイ (Gy)
放射能	ベクレル (Bq)
線量当量	シーベルト (Sv)

SI単位の因数，十進数表記の倍数と約数

増倍率	接頭辞	記号
10^{12}	テラ	T
10^9	ギガ	G
10^6	メガ	M
10^3	キロ	k
10^2	ヘクト	h
10^1	デカ	da
10^{-1}	デシ	d
10^{-2}	センチ	c
10^{-3}	ミリ	m

10^{-6}	micro	µ
10^{-9}	nano	n
10^{-12}	pico	p
10^{-15}	femto	f
10^{-18}	atto	A

Rules for using units and writing large numbers and decimals

—The symbol for a unit is unaltered in the plural and should not be followed by a full stop/point except at the end of a sentence: i.e. 2 cm, not 2 cm. or 2 cms.
—Large numbers are written in three-digit groups (working from right to left) with spaces not commas (in some countries the comma is used to indicate a decimal point): e.g. forty thousand is written as 40 000, four-hundred thousand is written as 400 000.
—Numbers with four numbers are written without the space: e.g. six thousand is written as 6000.
—The decimal sign between numbers is indicated by a full stop/point placed near the line: e.g. 40.75. If the numerical value of the decimal is less than 1, a zero should appear before the decimal sign: i.e. 0.125, not .125.
—Decimals with more than four numbers are also written in three-digit groups, but this time working from left to right: e.g. 0.000 25.
—'Squared' and 'cubed' are expressed as numerical powers and not by abbreviation: e.g. square centimetre is cm^2, not sq. cm.

10^{-6}	マイクロ	μ
10^{-9}	ナノ	n
10^{-12}	ピコ	p
10^{-15}	フェムト	f
10^{-18}	アト	A

単位の使用ならびに大数と小数の表記の規則

—単位の記号は複数形でも変化せず，文章の終わりを除きピリオドまたは点は付けない：例，2 cm. あるいは 2 cms. とせず 2 cm とする。

—大数は 3 桁ごとに分け (右から左に進む)，コンマではなくスペース (コンマが小数点を表すものとして使われている国もある) を入れて表記される。例：4 万は 40 000，40 万は 400 000 と表記される。

—4 桁はスペースなしで表記される。例：6 千は 6000。

—数字と数字の間の小数点の符号は，下付きのピリオドまたは点で表される：例，40.75。もし少数の数値が 1 より小さい場合には，0 を小数点の前に置く。例：0.125 であり .125 とは表記しない。

—4 桁より多い小数点も 3 桁ごとに表記されるが，この場合は左から右に進む。例：0.000 25。

—「2 乗」と「3 乗」は略語ではなく累乗の数値で表される。例：平方センチメートルは cm2 で sq. cm とは表記しない。

Commonly used measurements requiring further explanation

— *Volume:* volume is calculated by multiplying length, width and depth. Using the SI unit for length, the metre (m), means ending up with a cubic metre (m^3), which is a huge volume and it is not appropriate for most uses. In clinical practice the litre (L or l) is used. A litre is based on the volume of a cube measuring 10 cm × 10 cm × 10 cm. Smaller units still, e.g. Millilitre (mL) or one-thousandth of a litre, are commonly used in clinical practice.

— *Pressure:* the SI unit of pressure is the pascal (Pa), and the kilopascal (kPa) replaces the old non-SI unit of millimetres of mercury pressure (mmHg) for blood pressure and blood gases. However, mmHg are still widely used for measuring blood pressure. Other anomalies include: cerebrospinal fluid, which is measured in millimetres of water (mmH_2O); and central venous pressure, which is measured in centimetres of water (cmH_2O).

— *Temperature:* although the SI base unit for temperature is the kelvin, by international convention temperature is measured in degrees Celsius (°C).

— *Energy:* the energy of food or individual requirements for energy are measured in kilojoules (kJ); the SI unit is the joule (J). In practice, many people still use the kilocalorie (kcal), a non-SI unit, for these uses. 1 calorie = 4.2 J; 1 kilocalorie (large Calorie) = 4.2 kJ.

— *Time:* the SI base unit for time is the second (s), but it is acceptable to use minute (min), hour (h) or day (d). In clinical practice it is preferable to use 'per 24 hours' for the excretion of substances in urine and faeces: i.e. g/24 h.

— *Amount of substance:* the SI base unit for amount of substance is the mole (mol). The concentration of many substances is expressed in moles per litre (mol/L) or millimoles per litre (mmol/L), which replaces milliequivalents per litre (mEq/L). Some exceptions exist and include: haemoglobin and plasma proteins, which are given in grams per litre (g/L); and enzyme activity, which is given in International Units (IU, U or iu).

詳しい説明が必要な，良く使われる計量法

―*体積*：長さ，幅，奥行を掛けて求められる。長さを表す SI 単位，メートル（m）を使うということは，結局は立方メートル（m³）で表すということになる。これは非常に大きい容量であり，ほとんどの使用に適さない。臨床業務ではリットル（L または l）が使われる。リットルは 10 cm × 10 cm × 10 cm の立方体の体積を基にしている。ミリリットル（mL）すなわち 1 リットルの 1000 分の 1 のような，より小さい単位が今でも臨床実務で一般的に使われている。

―*圧力*：圧力の SI 単位はパスカル（Pa），キロパスカル（kPa）であり，血圧や血液ガスを表す，古い非 SI 単位の水銀柱ミリメートル（mmHg）に代わるものである。しかしながら，今でも水銀柱ミリメートルは血圧を計測するのに広く使われている。他にも例外として，水柱ミリメートル（mmH₂O）で計測される脳脊髄液，センチメートル水柱で計測される中心静脈圧などもある。

―*温度*：温度の SI 基本単位はケルビンだが，国際協定では，温度は摂氏温度で計測される。

―*エネルギー*：食物エネルギーや個々人のエネルギー所要量はキロジュール（kJ）で計測される。SI 単位はジュール（J）である。実際には，多くの人はまだこれらの用途に非 SI 単位のキロカロリー（kcal）を使っている。1 カロリー = 4.2 ジュール，1 キロカロリー（大カロリー）= 4.2 キロジュールである。

―*時間*：時間の SI 基本単位は秒（s）だが，分（min），時間（h）または日（d）も使うことができる。臨床実務では尿や便による物質の排出には「24 時間当たり」が好まれる。例：g/24 h（24 時間当たりのグラム数）。

―*物質量*：物質量の SI 基本単位はモル（mol）である。多くの物質の濃度はモル濃度（mol/L）あるいはミリモル濃度（mmol/L）で表され，ミリグラム当量（mEq/L）に代わるものである。いくつか例外も見られ，グラム毎リットル（g/L）で示されるヘモグロビンや血漿タンパク質，国際単位（IU，U または iu）で示される酵素活性などがある。

MEASUREMENTS, EQUIVALENTS AND CONVERSIONS (SI OR METRIC AND IMPERIAL)

Volume

1 litre (L) = 1000 millilitres (mL)
1 millilitre (mL) = 1000 microlitres (µL)

Note: The millilitre (mL) and the cubic centimetre (cm^3) are usually treated as being equivalent.

Conversions

1 litre (L) = 1.76 pints (pt)
568.25 millilitres (mL) = 1 pint (pt)
28.4 millilitres (mL) = 1 fluid ounce (fl oz)

Length

1 kilometre (km) = 1000 metres (m)
1 metre (m) = 100 centimetres (cm) or 1000 millimetres (mm)
1 centimetre (cm) = 10 millimetres (mm)
1 millimetre (mm) = 1000 micrometres (µm)
1 micrometre (µm) = 1000 nanometres (nm)

Conversions

1 metre (m) = 39.370 inches (in)
1 centimetre (cm) = 0.3937 inches (in)
30.48 centimetres (cm) = 1 foot (ft)
2.54 centimetres (cm) = 1 inch (in)

度量法，等価量，そして換算 (SI 単位，メートル法，そして英国度量衡法)

体積

1 リットル (L) = 1000 ミリリットル (mL)
1 ミリリットル (mL) = 1000 マイクロリットル (μL)

注：ミリリットル (mL) と平方センチメートル (cm^3) は通常等価として扱われる。

換算

1 リットル (L) = 1.76 パイント (pt)
568.25 ミリリットル (mL) = 1 パイント (pt)
28.4 ミリリットル (mL) = 1 液量オンス (fl oz)

長さ

1 キロメートル (km) = 1000 メートル (m)
1 メートル (m) = 1000 センチメートル (cm)
　　　　　　　または，1000 ミリメートル (mm)
1 センチメートル (cm) = 10 ミリメートル (mm)
1 ミリメートル (mm) = 1000 マイクロメートル (μm)
1 マイクロメートル (μm) = 1000 ナノメートル (nm)

換算

1 メートル (m) = 39.370 インチ (in)
1 センチメートル (cm) = 0.397 (in)
30.48 センチメートル (cm) = 1 フット (ft)
2.54 センチメートル (cm) = 1 インチ (in)

Weight or mass

1 kilogram (kg) = 1000 grams (g)
1 gram (g) = 1000 milligrams (mg)
1 milligram (mg) = 1000 micrograms (µg)
1 microgram (µg) = 1000 nanograms (ng)

Note: To avoid any confusion with milligram (mg) the word microgram (µg) should be written in full on prescriptions.

Conversions

1 kilogram (kg) = 2.204 pounds (1b)
1 gram (g) = 0.0353 ounce (oz)
453.59 grams (g) = 1 pound (1b)
28.34 grams (g) = 1 ounce (oz)

Temperature conversions

To convert Celsius to Fahrenheit, multiply by 9, divide by 5, and add 32 to the result. For example, to convert 36°C to Fahrenheit:

36 × 9 = 324 ÷ 5 = 64.8 + 32 = 96.8°F

therefore 36°C = 96.8°F.

To convert Fahrenheit to Celsius, subtract 32, multiply by 5, and divide by 9. For example, to convert 104°F to Celsius:

104 - 32 = 72 × 5 = 360 ÷ 9 = 40°C

therefore 104°F = 40°C.

重さまたは質量

1 キログラム (kg) = 1000 グラム (g)
1 グラム (g) = 1000 ミリグラム (mg)
1 ミリグラム (mg) = 1000 マイクログラム (μg)
1 マイクログラム (μg) = 1000 ナノグラム (ng)

*注：*ミリグラム (mg) との混同を避けるため，処方箋ではマイクログラム (μg) という単語は略さないで書かれるべきである。

換算

1 キログラム (kg) = 2.204 ポンド (lb)
1 グラム (g) = 0.035 オンス (oz)
453.59 グラム (g) = 1 ポンド (lb)
28.34 グラム (g) = 1 オンス (oz)

温度の換算

摂氏を華氏に換算するには，摂氏の温度に 9 を掛けたものを 5 で割り，出た数字に 32 を足す。例えば，36℃ を華氏にするには：

$$36 \times 9 = 324 \div 5 = 64.8 + 32 = 96.8°F$$

よって，36℃ = 96.8°F となる。

華氏を摂氏に換算するには，華氏の温度から 32 を引き，5 を掛けて 9 で割る。例えば，104°F を摂氏に換算するには：

$$104 - 32 = 72 \times 5 = 360 \div 9 = 40℃$$

よって，104°F = 40℃ となる。

Temperature comparison

°Celsius	°Fahrenheit
100	212
95	203
90	194
85	185
80	176
75	167
70	158
65	149
60	140
55	131
50	122
45	113
44	112.2
43	109.4
42	107.6
41	105.8
40	104
39.5	103.1
39	102.2
38.5	101.3
38	100.4
37.5	99.5
37	98.6
36.5	97.7
36	96.8

温度の比較

摂氏℃	華氏℉
100	212
95	203
90	194
85	185
80	176
75	167
70	158
65	149
60	140
55	131
50	122
45	113
44	112.2
43	109.4
42	107.6
41	105.8
40	104
39.5	103.1
39	102.2
38.5	101.3
38	100.4
37.5	99.5
37	98.6
36.5	97.7
36	96.8

35.5	95.9
35	95
34	93.2
33	91.4
32	89.6
31	87.8
30	86
25	77
20	68
15	59
10	50
5	41
0	32
-5	23
-10	14

Note:

Boiling point = 100°C = 212°F

Freezing point = 0°C = 32°F

FURTHER READING

Gatford JD, Phillips N 2002 Nursing calculations, 6th edn. Churchill Livingstone, Edinburgh.

35.5	95.9
35	95
34	93.2
33	91.4
32	89.6
31	87.8
30	86
25	77
20	68
15	59
10	50
5	41
0	32
-5	23
-10	14

注：

沸点 = 100℃ = 212°F

冰点 = 0℃ = 32°F

参考文献

Gatford JD, Phillips N 2002 Nursing calculations, 6th edn. Churchill Livingstone, Edinburgh.

● 著者

Joy Parkinson BA
Author and Lecturer,
Former Head of English,
Southwark College, London, UK

Chris Brooker BSc, MSc, RGN, SCM, RNT
Author and Lecturer, Norfolk, UK

● 訳者略歴

西村　月満（にしむらつきまろ）
慶應義塾大学大学院文学研究科博士課程修了
米国ウィスコンシン大学大学院修士課程修了（M. A. in English）
北里大学一般教育部元教授　専門：応用言語学、English for Specific Purposes、英語教育学
主な著書：*The Wonders of Medicine*（共著、南雲堂）、『21世紀のESP：英語教育学大系第4巻』（共著、大修館書店）、*Understanding Health Care*（共著、朝日出版社）、『日本医学英語検定試験3・4級教本』（共著、メジカルビュー社）、『薬学英語入門』（共著、東京化学同人）他。

平井　清子（ひらいせいこ）
津田塾大学学芸学部英文学科 卒業
米国フェアフィールド大学大学院修士課程修了（M. A. in Education）
北里大学一般教育部教授　専門：二言語習得研究、第二言語喪失研究、英語教育学
主な著書：『第二言語習得—SLA研究と外国語教育：英語教育学大系第5巻』（共著、大修館書店）、『レナードの朝で学ぶアメリカの医療と生活』（単著、南雲堂フェニックス）、『日本のバイリンガル教育—学校の事例から学ぶー』（共著、三修社）、『医療・看護・歯科英語基本用語用例集』（共著、南雲堂フェニックス）他。

和治元　義博（わじもとよしひろ）
学習院大学大学院人文科学研究科博士後期課程修了
北里大学一般教育部准教授　専門：中世英国演劇
主な著書：*The Wonders of Medicine*（共著、南雲堂）、*The Hospital Team — English for Medical Specialists*（共著、南雲堂）、『薬学英語基本用語用例集』（共著、南雲堂フェニックス）他。

著作権法上、無断複写・複製は禁じられています。

英和対訳　実践　看護の英会話

	2013年4月24日	1刷
著　者 —	ジョイ・パーキンスン	Joy Parkinson
	クリス・ブルッカー	Chris Brooker
訳注者 —	西村 月満	Tsukimaro Nishimura
	平井 清子	Seiko Hirai
	和治元 義博	Yoshihiro Wajimoto
発行者 —	南雲 一範	
発行所 —	株式会社 南雲堂	

〒162-0801　東京都新宿区山吹町 361
TEL　03-3268-2311　　FAX　03-3269-2486
振替　00160-0-4686
印刷所／日本ハイコム株式会社　　製本所／松村製本所
Printed in Japan　　乱丁・落丁本はお取り替えいたします。

ISBN978-4-523-26515-3　　C0082　　　　　　　　　　　[1-515]

E-mail　　nanundo@post.email.ne.jp
URL　　　http://www.nanun-do.co.jp